"As a psychologist who has worked for forty years with the disability population who require support from paid, professional staff I know that one of the most consistent challenges for people with disabilities and their families is to find caregivers who see "beyond the diagnosis," and who can relate to individuals as whole human beings with interests, needs, and personalities distinct from their disabilities. *Who Will Butter My Toast?* is an invaluable resource for professionals like me, and for the agencies and staff providing services. I highly recommend this heartfelt, personal, and well-written resource to anyone involved in a helping relationship."

Peter Love, MPH, PhD

"Although my son's challenges were far different than Sandy's daughter's, she had a deep understanding capturing my emotions. This same pathos shines through in *Who Will Butter My Toast?*—a true gem of a book for anyone hiring caregivers."

Amy Jaffe Barzach, *Accidental Courage, Boundless Dreams*, coauthored with Sandy Tovray Greenberg

"This guide is a must read for anyone who is caring for someone or who may be responsible for the task in the future. Sandy Greenberg provides a thorough, heartfelt book on what it takes as well as how to allow others to share in the process. She does not shy away from difficulties she has faced, and her advice on how to avoid potential challenges offers insights on how details in communication are critical for a team of people to work together. She gives a comprehensive set of directions on how to start the process, yet she also encourages you to be open to think about your own unique set of circumstances, and to incorporate them into her model."

Luisa DiNino-Jones, MSW, LMSW, CBIS, of Connecticut Community Care

"I was aware my mom's friend Sandy was writing a book about how to create a handbook for caregivers, but it wasn't until my mom broke her ankle that I truly gained an understanding of how valuable this resource is. She has recovered beautifully, but it opened my eyes to be more prepared for the future. The book is very well organized and detailed."

Stacy G, Operations Manager at a Boston Hospital

"Sandy's Handbook for Caregivers is an important resource for anyone with a family member who has a disability. Her thorough explanations and examples give readers a step-by-step guide to creating their own handbooks. I particularly appreciate that she keeps the individual with a disability at the center of the handbook. Too often well-meaning family and caregivers think they know best when caring for someone and forget that, in most cases, it is important to ask what the individual wants or needs. Thank you, Sandy, for sharing this important guide."

Julie Peters, CBIS, Executive Director, Brain Injury Alliance of Connecticut

Who Will Butter My Toast?

How to Create a Handbook for Caregivers

SANDY TOVRAY GREENBERG

Order this book online at www.trafford.com
or email orders@trafford.com

Most Trafford titles are also available at major online book retailers.

Print information available on the last page.

ISBN: 978-1-6987-1127-0 (sc)
ISBN: 978-1-6987-1128-7 (e)

Library of Congress Control Number: 2022903802

Trafford rev. 06/14/2023

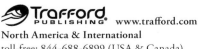 www.trafford.com

North America & International
toll-free: 844-688-6899 (USA & Canada)
fax: 812-355-4082

Dedication

To my daughter Rayna, my stop sign to relish the aroma of roses; and to my daughter Tovah, my rock who reminds me to choose happy in life; who both, for different reasons, are true heroes teaching and inspiring me each day.

To Richard, for his day-to-day loving support.

To caregivers everywhere, for whom we are forever grateful.

Contents

PART FOUR: RAYNA'S LEAD TEAM MEMBER HANDBOOK: SAMPLE

PART FIVE: RAYNA'S KEY FAMILY HANDBOOK: SAMPLE

Acknowledgments

The expression "It takes a village" also applies to creating this book. Thank you to all who gave feedback, assisted with editing, and provided helpful suggestions and support along the way. To Rayna and Tovah; my son-in-law, Carl Spring; my husband, Richard; Rayna's dad, Allyn; Nina B. Lichtenstein, my talented social media manager and editor; my childhood friends, Myra Glansberg and Roberta Chadis, who offered invaluable insight and have been so generous with their time and laughter as we deviated and reminisced; to Nancy Reese, Jemuel East and Leni Weintraub. I am also grateful to another special childhood friend, Sara Ganz, who listened with wide open ears, strong shoulders, and a caring heart as I talked endlessly about the book's progress; my good friend, Carmen Sanchez, for enthusiastically suggesting to use *Who Will Butter My Toast?* when I showed her my list of title possibilities, and I instantly realized all the other titles paled in comparison; to fellow writers, Nancy Manning and Denise Heroux McShane, who inspire me and cheer me on; and Rayna's extraordinary neuropsychologist, Dr. Peter Love, who offered keen insights I never would have imagined for this book in addition to his expertise in guiding Rayna. Thank you to Rayna's social worker over many years, Luisa DiNino-Jones of Connecticut Community Care, for her expertise in guiding me and "aligning the stars," and to all caregivers who gave feedback for this project. Thank you also to Nina, Richard, Tovah, along with my brother, Dr. Roy Steiman, and my cousin, Barbara Rozavsky, for all their creative suggestions for the book cover. Thank you to Laura Ernst, Rayna's physical therapist, for her guidance in how best to describe directives related to my daughter's mobility and safety.

I am also grateful to the states where Rayna has resided, home state of Massachusetts, Florida, Connecticut, and New Jersey, and to every stellar person and organization who help Rayna live a safe and happy life.

Thank you to all those at Trafford Publishing, who helped polish and prepare my manuscript to ready it for the world.

Message from the Author

I wrote this book based on personal experiences, love, compassion, and many years of robust involvement as the mother of a child with special needs. Love and compassion, the foundation of my world. Love for Rayna, and love for Tovah, who took on the title of "special sibling" and relentlessly showers her little sister (and me) with caring support; love for every family member, friend, and professional who has been an integral part of Rayna's life.

From the challenges I have faced and my learning curve over all the years that I have worked with my daughter's caregivers, I have garnered useful insights to help you create a handbook for your loved one, whether an elderly relative, a child with a disability, a close friend, etc.

After Rayna's brain bleed at age three, we coordinated our daughter's care and activities throughout her childhood and teens. When she was in her late twenties, she began living on her own with assistance from the state of Connecticut Acquired Brain Injury Waiver. I handed over the day-to-day reins to professional caregivers while serving as her care coordinator. Well, I didn't quite hand over those reins, but I learned to loosen them a little. As they say, always a mother. And because Rayna's disability involves memory issues, I am often her spokesperson.

A simple question from Rayna when she first acquired caregivers became my driving force for developing a handbook. "Mommy, can you tell caregivers not to put their pocketbooks on my kitchen table or couch? They can be dirty."

So caregivers were informed of Rayna's request. Asked, answered, and done, until soon after, another situation arose when I discovered unlabeled tuna salad in Rayna's refrigerator, which made it difficult to know whether it was safe to eat without contacting caregivers who worked in the past few days. Now I needed to remember two requests: pocketbook location and food labeling.

Rayna's simple question planted a seed as more and more directives popped into my mind. I should tell caregivers about this, remind them about that, let them know how to . . . I started a list. I realized that while these caring people were skilled, they did not know how Rayna, with the help of family, preferred to run her household, not necessarily like their households or those of other households. The more I wrote, the more ideas sprouted to keep Rayna safe, happy, and living a dignified life in a smoothly run home. I found comfort in putting these directives in writing; Rayna's preferences of how she likes her chicken cooked, making sure to label leftovers, what music she likes, rules to help her be safe, medical directives, pillows arranged on her bed to best help her right-sided weakness, and more. A lot to remember and share.

The list grew and grew and grew. I decided to categorize topics. Pocketbook request went under general caregiver rules; leftovers labeling belonged on a kitchen list. I added new topics: keeping track of medical information, laundry, going out in the community, etc.

As life progressed, so did information that needed to be communicated to caregivers. Lists begat sections; sections begat chapters; chapters begat table of contents. From Rayna's initial request about pocketbooks came the birth of a handbook.

And that birth eventually brought forth an epiphany that if this handbook is valuable for Rayna's care, wouldn't other families of loved ones be able to benefit from my ideas and use the lessons I learned on this caregiving journey? That's when I decided to morph Rayna's handbook into a how-to book; to teach families and friends of loved ones with special and/or aging needs steps in creating a handbook for caregivers, using Rayna's and my experiences as an example.

In addition to Rayna's pocketbook request planting a seed for creating a handbook, she also inspired the title for this how-to book. Because her right side is partially paralyzed, she requires help with many tasks. When Rayna was younger, long before leaving home and living on her own, and long before the word "caregivers" was on my radar screen, I was filing her nails. As we sat side by side, I held her hand, and she asked, "Mommy, who will file my nails when I am older?"

That question resonated with me, and I surmised, without being truly aware of her intentions, that she was also asking who would take care of her as she reached adulthood and even when I am no longer here. I deduced that this question might be the first in a long line of many others as she grew. "Who will help me put on mittens?" "Who will teach me how to dress my doll?" "Who will butter my toast?" As Rayna's mother, I also pondered her future. Who *will* butter her toast?

Many times, as I undertook this project to create a handbook to make sure Rayna will always be cared for in a manner she wants and we, as her loving family, strive to achieve for her,

I experienced a sensation these handbooks were part of her legacy. Tovah has benevolently volunteered to oversee her sister's care in the future, and a step-by-step handbook will be a true asset to sustain Rayna's caregiving lineage. Even if you are writing a caregiver handbook for an elderly loved one, it can still be a legacy because no one knows what fate brings us. Whatever your circumstances—large family, small family, friends to help, or even if none of these options are available—having a handbook can also be a type of legacy for your loved one.

I know my handbook has greatly diminished angsts for Rayna's current and future caregiving, and if I can do the same for you, I will have accomplished something worthwhile.

Part One

How to Create a
Handbook for Caregivers

Section A

Introduction

Before we begin, a little housekeeping for *Who Will Butter My Toast?*

- Caregivers are referred to as "she" or "her" because we only employ female caregivers for Rayna's home.
- For parts 1 and 2, all Rayna's team members and lead team member are referred to as caregiver or lead caregiver.
- For parts 3, 4, and 5, the sample handbooks, caregiver is replaced with TM (team member or members) and lead caregiver is replaced with LTM (lead team member). Why? Because once caregivers are hired, these are the terms we use.

House is cleaned. Let's move on!

Start by building your handbook with the foundation: terminology.

Handbook versus Guide versus Manual versus Booklet

A slight difference but worth noting:

Handbook:	Usually a topically organized book for a certain location and purpose
Manual:	Addresses more about instructions, such as assembling a product
Guidebook:	May also be a manual yet usually teaches in quicker steps
Booklet:	A little book

Caretaker versus Caregiver

I never knew differences existed between these words until I researched them.

- Caregiver typically refers to an individual giving physical and emotional support to people.
- Caretaker, albeit still referring to caring for a person, can also be used for a place or thing, such as lawn care.

Slight difference. Your choice of words.

For your handbook, you can continue to use terms such as "caregiver," "caretaker," "staff," "employee," or "team member" as we do for Rayna's caregivers.

Title for Lead Caregiver

- Select, when possible, one person to be a lead caregiver whether within the slate of caregivers hired or an outside person.
  - Identify this person with a title.
  - Suggestions include "lead caregiver," "lead team member," "lead staff," "key staff," and "house manager."
  - The agency we use selects one of Rayna's team members who is referred to as "lead team member," so we mirror that word in the handbook. More about agencies and lead caregiver position in part 2.

Title for Contact Person

- When possible, families should select a contact person to act as a representative or liaison and be responsible to disseminate all information to family members and caregivers.
- Identify a backup or as many backups as possible.
  - I like to identify this person by a title rather than surname. I use "key family." Other suggestions include "liaison," "key contact," "main family," "main contact."
    - In some situations, there may be no family member to step in, so perhaps a friend, lawyer, social worker, or another professional could accept this role. Suggestions for this title include "key contact" or "key friend."
  - More about key contact position in part 2.
- Be consistent with titles—for example, if you opt for "key family," stay with "key family"; do not interchange terms such as sometimes writing "main family."

Terminology in place. Now onto why a handbook. This handbook is to be helpful in numerous situations:

- You are responsible for your loved one's care.
- You may have been asked or volunteered to accept a caregiving position.
- You may have an employment situation or not live geographically close or other circumstances may prevent you from being a daily hands-on caregiver.
- You are starting a search for caregivers.
- You have already secured caregivers yet need more guidance.

No matter the scenario, it's never too early to start thinking about what information caregivers should know to keep your loved one's life running as smoothly and safely as possible. How many times have you asked a multitude of questions? "Who will know how to . . . ?" "Who will be able to . . . when I am not here?" "Who will do . . . ?" Or you might counter, "I am my loved one's caregiver and know her best and everything she needs." Yet what if you need an extra hand when you can't be there? Even if you engaged backups, how will your loved one's needs be conveyed?

Suppose you were bringing your loved one to a doctor but ran into a last-minute glitch. Even if you were able to find someone to step in, how do you effectively impart all the necessary information to your last-minute savior, such as

- doctor's name and address,
- number to call if they hit traffic and run late,
- necessary documents to bring to this appointment,
- questions to ask the doctor,
- cell phone numbers,
- explanations of safety precautions, and
- medications needed when out in the community.

These few examples are for one situation. Many other day-to-day details exist. What about food? Will your loved one's home be filled with her favorite foods? What are they? You tell a caregiver, "She likes . . ." Then the next time this caregiver works, your "She likes . . ." changed to "Oh, and she doesn't seem to like . . .," and you need to remember to communicate that new information. Remembering every detail to help your loved one stay safe and happy is challenging. Having procedures, lists, instructions, and communication systems in place will help enable continuity of care for other caregivers to follow.

Accepting your loved one needs caregiving might make you feel anxious. Giving up any portion of control can be scary yet can also bring relief. I get it. When you turn over the reins or even share those reins for your loved one's care, even if temporary, think how much smoother the transition will be when you have a handbook in place.

Keep in mind, a handbook for caregivers that details every aspect of day-to-day living is not a one-size fits all. No two handbooks will ever be identical. A wide range of specific needs exists for each individual needing care. Yours may include a

- handbook only for physical and mental health information, or only medical information, or any combination;
- handbook of five pages, fifty-five pages, or any number of pages;
- handbook dictated by number of hours needed;
- handbook dictated by number of caregivers needed;
- handbook for lead caregiver services and/or key family, if those positions are ideal for you; and
- handbook that includes apartment or congregant housing rules, if applicable.

Thus, as requirements for caregiving vary, so too will your handbook. Your situations for caregiving needs might be similar or have no resemblance to my samples. You may not need to include certain directives that are in my handbook yet should include specific instructions based on *your* loved one's needs.

Your instructions for pill-taking might only need something like, "Give daily pills in morning." For Rayna's daily pills, after caregivers assist Rayna to pour them in a little cup, they cannot simply place the pill cup next to her and walk away. Because of Rayna's memory challenges, she may forget to take them even with a filled cup sitting next to her, so caregivers must cue her and watch her take the pills. Thus, a different directive in the handbook.

Although the core of this book instructs how to create a handbook for caregivers, I want to briefly address finding caregivers either through an agency or private help. A world of support to secure caregivers is available from many sources, including

- websites with topics such as elderly, disability, homecare agencies, and caregiving;
- websites from federal, state, and town governments;
- reference books;
- organizations of generalized populations such as the elderly;
- organizations of specific disabilities, such as brain injury, MS, stroke, etc.;
- Facebook groups;
- civic organizations;

- medical professionals, social workers; and
- teachers, friends, and family.

Having a child with a disability, I have great appreciation of all who have helped our family enable Rayna to live on her own, including medical professionals, friends, relatives, numerous caregivers, and the state agencies for providing services that she needs as an adult living independently. We have had a bevy of caregivers who deserve accolades for their extraordinary dedication in caring for and loving our daughter, and I am deeply grateful for them and respect their crucial role. I want to wrap them in gold paper with big shiny bows because they are true gifts. Yet a bruised apple occasionally slips in. My advice is to keep your eyes wide open.

Look for red flags such as

- theft,
- abuse (verbal and/or physical),
- negligence,
- caregiver who is uncooperative,
- caregiver with a negative attitude,
- caregiver who doesn't follow established procedures, and
- caregiver who is not a team player.

We haven't experienced everything on this list, yet we've had some disturbing incidents. Some homes even install nanny cams, and if you do, be sure to comply with the laws for using such devices.

Never assume—everything is possible. Erase this thought: "No one would ever do that in my loved one's home." However, do not let this warning deter you from the ultimate good caregivers provide. Before seeking out a caregiver(s) or hiring an agency to provide a caregiver(s), research as much as possible. Many websites offer information for interviewing applicants, background checks, gathering references, and so forth that you should always address.

If you realize that the agency you selected isn't a good fit, shop around for others. This has happened with Rayna's care.

Final thoughts before moving on to section B, "Preparation." There is only one you, and you can't be replaced. A set of instructions helps ensure your loved one's safety and care in your absence.

Section B

Preparation

Before creating a handbook for caregivers, I suggest following several steps.

Step 1: Mindset

Start by being assured that once completed, your endeavors will result in a valuable tool to facilitate the care your loved one needs and deserves. Remove words such as "overwhelming" or "daunting" from your creating-a-handbook vocabulary and mindset. Keep "patient" and "determined."

I model the following motivations about reassurance and being patient:

> A writing teacher once asked our class whether we can move a large boulder. A roar of "no" reverberated. "Can you move a stone?" A roar of "yes" was returned. He encouraged us to think of our writing as chiseling one stone off the boulder, move it, chisel another stone, add that stone to the first one, and repeat this process until a boulder has been moved. If you mirror this approach, one stone at a time, you will have eventually moved your boulder, written your handbook.

> As seen on a billboard posting for a large construction project in Boston:
> "Rome wasn't built in a day—If it were, we would have hired their contractors."

Facing the challenges of caregiving with patience will be beneficial. Many emotions are involved in your experiences with caregivers; however, to keep grounded, consider caregiving as administrative responsibilities. Take off your emotional hat and put on a business hat. In a sense, taking care of a loved one with the help of caregivers is like running a small business. A handbook helps avoid preventable problems and will make life easier for everyone. By being patient and understanding that creating your handbook is a process of collecting, organizing, and communicating information, you are on your way to success.

You do not need to undertake this project alone. There are many resources to help you create a handbook, so keep "support" in your mindset.

- Read my sample handbooks in parts 3, 4, and 5 as a springboard to get started and to reference as you create your own.
- Reach out to friends and family for input.
- Consult with your loved one's roster of professionals, including neuropsychologists, physical and occupational therapists, psychologists, social workers, and medical doctors. Their expertise and perspectives are invaluable.
- Reach out to caregivers for ideas.
- If possible, reach out to one more person who might benefit from being involved in determining what caregiving is needed—your loved one!

One final preparation suggestion: After you take off your emotional hat, try to keep it off as much as possible.

Step 2: Technology

Part of preparation includes setting up folders and Word documents.

- Create one main folder on your computer. I recommend labeling it the title of your handbook. This folder should include two sub folders: Active and Backup.
  - Active (for the draft you are currently working on)
    - Word documents, one for each chapter of the handbook—for example, "Safety," "Laundry," "Kitchen," "Bedtime." Creating handbook chapters on separate Word documents makes for easier updating.
    - One Word document for notes and ideas about what to include in the handbook. I suggest you start capturing your ideas by evaluating your loved one's needs. I label this document "Extra Material."

  - Backup (for each draft you create in the editing and updating process)
    - I suggest dating every draft so that you never have to wonder which one is the most recent.

Step 3: Evaluate Loved One's Needs

When I taught a seminar on how to start a memoir, I suggested my students begin the process by simply writing their stories and not worrying about grammar, run-on sentences, or dotting i's and crossing t's at this point. The most crucial part is to capture an idea on paper before it's forgotten. Use this same approach with your handbook: capture ideas, organize them, and then fine-tune.

To evaluate your loved one's needs, observe her through the eyes of someone meeting her for the first time. Any observation can be valuable so another caregiver can step in.

- Think of broad topics you want communicated, such as medical information, finances, food, general household, chores, hygiene, taking your loved one out in the community, safety, emergency . . .
- Break down these broad topics into subheadings for more details.

The core of a comprehensive handbook is details, no matter how inconsequential they may seem. Remember, you want to communicate clearly.

Is a trip out in the community for social plans or a medical appointment? If some rules for going out in the community and returning home apply to both, introduce this topic with general details, and then branch out with specifics for social plans and specifics for medical appointments. Similarly, a safety chapter involves general safety information and then subtopics for physical, medical, emotional, and housing safety.

As you progress with your handbook, this list of needs will most likely grow and become more comprehensive. Simply add new revelations under the corresponding topic. As I was in the final stages of editing Rayna's latest edition of her handbook, an important point that had never dawned on me came to mind and was easily added to the appropriate chapter and section.

How to keep track of your ideas:

- Write directly into a Word document.
- Handwrite in a notebook or talk into a recording device and later transcribe all information to the Word document you created.

Be prepared for ideas to pop up at any time. I always take my "personal secretary," Siri, with me to record thoughts, especially when an OMG strikes me. "OMG, I didn't remind X about Y to . . ." "OMG, I didn't say . . ." "OMG, I forgot to explain how to . . ." "Siri! Remind me to add . . . to handbook."

Step 4: Assumptions to Awareness

Another word to remove from your vocabulary: assumptions. Assumptions are a forerunner to potential problems or, as I prefer, "hiccups." Assumptions transformed into awareness can result in less hiccups.

Caregivers, as superb as they can be in caregiving from training and experience, come to the position with perspectives based on their life experiences. Your vision of common knowledge is not necessarily in another person's wheelhouse. I assumed caregivers would automatically perform certain tasks the way we do them. This is not to be condescending. On the flipside, I have been unaware of valuable information Rayna's caregivers have shared with us—for example, some new cooking and cleaning tips.

Don't assume caregivers will know your preferences. Having information listed in a handbook ensures that everyone knows what procedures are to be followed. For example, if not told, how would they know your loved one's preferred way for food preparation is roasting and not frying?

We also embrace caregivers' backgrounds and family histories. Rayna loves to exchange information. They have swapped stories of their culture, holiday traditions, introduced new recipes (and have cooked some of their traditional dishes together), and so forth. At the same time, you need to set boundaries for information that you deem inappropriate to share. We have had caregivers disclose details about financial woes, legal problems, and intimate stories about boyfriends . . . These incidents led me to include a list of taboo subjects for sharing.

Frustrating as hiccups can be, I try to make them learning experiences to improve Rayna's care in the future. When this happens, I immediately use the opportunity to add, delete, or edit the handbook directive, which, in turn, lessens worries about Rayna. I understood her caregiving situation wasn't necessarily going to be perfect, but I was still motivated to make it as seamless as possible. As I became more aware of eliminating assumptions, I initiated many directives before a hiccup occurred. "An ounce of prevention is worth a pound of cure." This quote by Benjamin Franklin surely applied to creating these handbooks. Unfortunately, many assumptions led to many hiccups until I caught on to Franklin's wise words.

I am reminded of a story while interviewing Amy Jaffe Barzach, the coauthor of *Accidental Courage, Boundless Dreams*, a memoir about her conception to build a playground accessible to all in memory of her son, Jonathan. When we began working on her project, Amy remarked that she didn't know what she didn't know. I often think about that comment and how it applies to my situation. Some hiccups originated from assumptions; others came from learning by mistakes and others from not knowing what I didn't know.

Here are some assumptions and hiccups resulting in awareness and handbook entries:

- **Assumption: Caregivers never touch Rayna's electronics.**
- Hiccup: Caregivers used laptop without permission.
- Awareness: Lock laptop. Add note on top that it's only for lead caregiver and Rayna's use.

- **Assumption: No one would unlock Rayna's door.**
- Hiccup: Rayna's door locks automatically, yet I have a habit to check the doorknob whenever I leave her apartment. One morning, on a visit to Rayna, I found her door unlocked. Caregiver explained she ran to the laundry room, unlocked the door for a "quick minute," rather than take the key FOB[1] to get back into the apartment, and forgot about locking the door. Never would I have thought caregivers would do that and, to my dismay, discovered she wasn't the only one unlocking the door.
- Awareness: Amended a directive in the safety section in a chapter to never unlock door. To be extra cautious, I taped a large reminder note on Rayna's door. Can't assume; didn't know what I didn't know!

Some hiccups such as electronics and unlocked door were solved and done; others led to more detailed directives.

- **Assumption: Caregivers do laundry exactly how we did before Rayna lived on her own.**
- Hiccup: Jeans were put in dryer. We prefer jeans hung to dry to avoid possible shrinkage.
- Awareness 1: Directive in chapter with laundry section to hang jeans instead of putting in dryer.
- Awareness 2: Hiccup led me to question what other laundry procedures were not being followed, such as for bedding, which we wash on a hot setting. So another directive was added to the handbook about laundry temperature settings and other clothes not to put in dryer.

---

1 A key fob (FOB) is a small security device with built-in authentication used to control and secure access to locked doors, network services, and data.

- **Assumption: No one would put an item in a place other than where item was found.**
- Hiccup: One day Rayna couldn't find a favorite dress. We finally located it hanging in an obscure place. The caregiver explained that the dress was still damp when laundry was retrieved from the dryer, so she hung the dress aside to finish drying. Clever thought process; however, the problem was that she never told anyone!
- Awareness 1: Assigned locations for items and added directive to replace all items to those locations; otherwise, misplaced items can wreak havoc, causing angst to find lost items, and ultimately an unnecessary waste of time for all.
- Awareness 2: Notify caregivers we welcome suggestions for moving items in apartment. Ask first!

- **Assumption: Caregivers will ask for directions when something unexpected happens.**
- Hiccup: Caregiver found an item in a different location and continued using that new spot, again causing lost time searching for it.
- Awareness: Caregivers will be notified if we change location, and without such notice, a new location only indicates someone did not return the item to its proper place.

These examples represent some of the hiccups that have occurred over the years, resulting in disorganization and frustration. We have encountered more crucial issues like a misplaced lab slip for a blood test, which led to creating a system to designate places for caregivers, lead caregiver, and family for important documents and messages.

Sometimes hiccups came from assumptions and other times, such as finding Rayna's door unlocked, from an accidental discovery as a result of my habit to check her door. While we try to eliminate assumptions, we can't always predict what may happen. All we can do is record those learning moments into our handbook directives.

With awareness and experience, hiccups have waned. Don't assume. Be aware. Communicate.

Step 5: Getting Organized

Getting organized includes setting up

- caregivers,
- loved one's home, and
- communication systems.

Caregivers

Just as you observed your loved one as though you were meeting her for the first time, every word in your handbook should be written as though each caregiver *is* working for the very first time and knows nothing about your loved one and how the household is run. Each shift of each day has the potential of having a new or substitute caregiver.

Along with general daily procedures for all shifts, various chores are delegated to specific shifts—for example, laundry is assigned to specific times. Without this organization, caregivers might notice a filled laundry basket yet not realize doing laundry is her responsibility for that shift. By assigning tasks and procedures, a caregiver knows her responsibilities, and with the benefit of a handbook as a reference, she will also not put jeans in the dryer!

Although all caregivers must complete many chores and tasks, some may have preferred interests and stronger skills—for example, all caregivers are responsible for Rayna's meals, yet this does not preclude one great chef making her delicious recipes and freezing them for later use.

Setting up a weekly calendar to capitalize on caregivers' specialties provides better care and improves morale. If you use an agency that requires a certain agenda for their employees, work with them to balance ways you want caregivers to assume responsibilities.

Side Notes about New and Substitute Caregivers

I am not a lover of four-letter words, especially "subs"! And throw in a three-letter word, "new." I am referring to caregivers who are subs or new to the position, "first-shifters." Intellectually, I understand subs are necessary, and I have a great amount of gratitude for them. In fact, some of them even become permanent caregivers. And intellectually, I also understand subs and every new caregiver hired must start with a first shift. Yet my heart unintentionally puts new caregivers and subs in a category worse than nails on a chalkboard. When planned, this unfamiliar person may be trained in advance, and Rayna's agency arranges for a new employee to shadow a current caregiver, yet last-minute situations can happen.

Permanent caregivers know "everything" to take care of Rayna, and my comfort level increases with their longevity as I witness how well Rayna thrives when a caregiver is a "keeper." Then in walks a person, as superb and capable as she may be, who doesn't know "everything" and is not familiar with Rayna. Thus, the birth of an orientation sheet for first-shifters. Although I truly needed to work harder to put on my all-business hat and keep that emotional hat far away in creating this orientation sheet, my angst was greatly reduced. Details about an orientation sheet for first-shifters are in section C in this chapter.

Loved One's Home

Label every cabinet and drawer so caregivers can easily locate products and return them to the correct location.

One of the best ways to keep a home with caregivers running smoothly is to designate a section or sections for all communication materials to lessen chances of misplacements and to give caregivers quick access to materials.

1. Communication Center

Rayna's apartment has a long table we call "communication table," which consists of

- communication basket: holds clipboards and forms caregivers need to fill out;
- various binders, such as Food/Recipe binder and caregiver handbook;
- contacts/passwords book;
- desk organizer;
- mailboxes: a set of three drawers used for messages and important papers, one each for caregiver, lead caregiver, and key family; and
- orientation basket: holds orientation sheet.

2. Dining Table

The dining table, across from the communication table, is divided in two parts:

- left side: for Rayna to eat
- right side: for caregivers to write their communications and to join Rayna for meals

3. Various Walls

I assign numbers to various walls in the apartment where I hang up information that I want seen easily without needing to flip to a section in the handbook.

- Wall 1 has the corkboard/whiteboard reserved for messages and updates of a crucial event that happens on a caregiver's shift, like Rayna became sick or heard upsetting news, so that all incoming shifts clearly see this information.

- Wall 2 is closest to a recliner chair where Rayna likes to sit in the living room and where she lies back for her daily dry eye treatments, so that's where I tacked up instructions for this procedure.
- Wall 3 holds a variety of postings, such as laundry card sign-out form, list of fall-risk prevention steps, crisis sheet, emergency contacts, and a list of allergies and intolerances.

All the other walls? Reserved for family photos, artwork (including some of Rayna's pieces), volunteer of the year award and diploma from special needs college (summa cum laude!). After all, it is still her home.

Communication Systems

In creating modes of communication, an important concept to remember is flexibility. By trial and error over the years, I have developed various communication systems and strategies in attempts to keep Rayna's life safe, smooth, and happy.

If applicable, your handbook should address communication from

- caregivers to caregivers;
- caregivers to lead caregiver;
- lead caregiver to caregivers;
- lead caregiver to key family; and
- lead caregiver to agency, if using an agency.

I believe the core of communication is what I like to call a "put and get" rule:

- *Put* all communication in writing.
- *Get* initials on written communication, whether caregivers initiate or read a communication.

Put

- Never have a serious conversation or announce a change without notifying caregivers in writing.
- If you unexpectedly need to relay information verbally, send a follow-up e-mail to confirm caregivers understood your communication, as well as to ensure a paper trail in case of a glitch.

Get

- Beyond accountability, signing communications also serves to know when a caregiver has read them, so you can remove the notice from the mailbox.
- Ask caregivers to print clearly.
- If the communication is to all caregivers, I include an "initial strip" at the bottom requesting they all sign and return form to caregiver mailbox, where it remains until all caregivers have read and initialed communication.
- Initial strip looks like this:

I have read this communication.

Initial: _____ _____ _____ _____ _____ _____ _____

Rayna's handbook samples include more information about communication forms.

If a communication form isn't working, make changes. Bank old system in your backup folder. You may later decide one part of that system could still work and simply needs tweaking. When I discovered a chart or form wasn't effective or was confusing to follow, I redesigned it. Try, try again, is the mantra!

Rayna has a witty sense of humor, and after several times hearing me explain a new communication form to caregivers, she once piped up, "Don't get used to this. My mom will change it." We should remember humor amid challenges!

Along with forms for caregivers to fill out and/or read, key family may want to initiate a regular newsletter (weekly, biweekly, monthly, or whatever time frame you think necessary).

A newsletter can

- offer good and welfare;
- congratulate and wish good luck to caregivers who experience a special event;
- express condolences if caregiver suffered a loss;
- share news about your loved one, a new accomplishment, announcement of a special occasion or any event in your loved one's life or family, such as a wedding or graduation;
- announce launch of finished handbook;
- announce a handbook change and include the edits.

Recapitulation of Preparation Steps

Now that you have adopted a mindset to be patient and not overwhelmed, scrapped assumptions, created Word documents and folders to organize your information, begun assessing your loved one's needs, organized forms, assigned locations for caregivers' communication needs, and hung up your emotional hat, you are already on the road to creating your caregiver handbook! Let's do this!

Creating a Caregiver Handbook

While you create a handbook, you may have a situation that needs immediate attention and can't wait until your handbook is completed. Case in point, the onset of Covid-19, which led me to create a list of Rayna-specific guidelines in addition to those the CDC and our agency put forth. Most of these extra guidelines were emotionally oriented because of Rayna's cognitive level. I designed a Covid-19 sheet and posted it in the apartment.

- My Covid sheet led me to realize that in creating my handbook directives about safety and addressing emotional issues, I never thought of a major crisis. So I created a crisis sheet.
- I address any type of crisis as well as steps to help Rayna if she hears upsetting news.
- For each crisis, I simply amend the information to match the current situation.

Creating Chapters

- Set up separate Word documents for each chapter.
- Title each chapter for broad categories to organize information.
- Your chapters and titles may change as you progress.
  - "Laundry" originally was a separate chapter, yet as I edited and tightened information, "Laundry" ended up with much fewer pages and was combined with the "Food and Household" chapter, and that even morphed later into one large chapter titled "Daily Procedures."
- Divide chapters into subtopics and title them "Sections" to make it easier to find information.
- I title sections using letters—for example, "Laundry" would be in chapter 4, "Daily Procedures," section C.

Suggestion to Layout of Handbook

1. Title page
2. Orientation
3. Table of contents
4. How to read handbook (you may also put some of this information in orientation)
   - Explain names of people and initials that you selected for a lead caregiver, main contact, etc. (discussed in terminology in section A, "Introduction").
   - Explain any special layout of handbook.
5. Chapters

A Detour Back to Orientation

Ideas for your first-shifters orientation sheet:

- Include a warm welcome from family and/or loved one and express your appreciation.
- Include highlights of most crucial information from your caregiver handbook to carry them through a first shift.
- Protect in a plastic sleeve.
- Put sheet in a basket and designate a place to keep that basket in the communication area of your loved one's home.
- Copy and place in front of the handbook as an extra precaution in case a caregiver accidentally misplaces the sheet.

Although an outgoing caregiver is more than happy to share information with an incoming first-shifter, that caregiver may need to leave immediately for another commitment when her shift ends. So in my quest to try to turn over every caregiving stone, I designed an order to the arrival of a first-shifter.

1. I created a sign:
   - top line: "Welcome to Rayna's Home!"
   - bottom line: "If this is your first shift, instructions are in basket labeled 'Orientation Basket' and located on long table behind living room chairs."
2. I placed the orientation sheet in the basket, which directs the first-shifter to the handbook.
3. I posted the sign on Rayna's door.

I liken my system to a treasure hunt with each clue leading to placing a first-shifter in a better position to take care of my loved one, who, after all, is a treasure! Door sign leads to orientation basket that leads to handbook and leads to better chances of a successful first shift.

Writing Styles

- Write topic and then explain details underneath.
- Be very detailed. The more specific, the less chance of derailment and hiccups.
- Use bullet points to organize directives.
- Use short sentences when possible.
- Be clear.
  - When choosing words, ask yourself what you are trying to convey and in what tone.
  - Omit subjective words, such as "occasional," "about," "small," or "large." These words lead to individual interpretations that might not result in what you want or your loved one needs.
  - If you want your loved one to follow a diet dictated by a particular portion control, don't say "small amount"—specify portion size, such as half-cup.
  - Be direct—don't imply and hope your wording will be correctly interpreted. If you mean "should," write "should"; if you mean "must," write "must"; if you mean "never," write "never."
  - Keep in mind there are exceptions. Do your best to adhere to exact words.

Section D

Editing

You completed a first draft. Congratulations! Now it's time to edit—an extremely crucial step in creating your handbook. And not only by you . . . many eyes lead to deeper vision. You can opt to seek readers after your first draft or when you feel you are finished after many drafts and ready for new eyes to look at your handbook.

Before You Edit

- Copy and paste original draft into a new Word document that now becomes draft 1.
- Choose an easy-to-recognize title for your drafts to be edited because you will probably have more than one draft as you continue to edit.
- Examples of titles:
  - dates: "HandbookOct12," "HandbookNov15," and so forth
  - numbers: "Handbook1," "Handbook2," and so forth
  - initials: "Loved One Caregiver Handbook" would be "LOCH" and backup titles: "LOCH1," "LOCH2" or "LOCHOct12," "LOCHNov15," and so forth
- Place this draft in your backup folder that you set up in technology step, in preparing to create the handbook.
- Now start editing what is draft 2. Keep this draft in your active file.
- Each time you edit, repeat the process, keep active draft until you are ready to edit, and then copy, put in backup folder, start a new Word document, paste, and title.
- For extra safety put your documents on an external hard drive, and/or e-mail them to yourself.
- Enjoy a level of comfort by knowing your original document and each draft are securely saved in several places. So edit away—add, delete, change.

When You Are Ready for Readers

My many readers included professionals, friends, family, including Rayna herself. And because I already had caregivers while writing the handbook, many of them gave feedback.

Some helped with certain sections and some for all the books, and each provided help in different ways. You may choose editing a few drafts with only one person reading at a time because multiple feedbacks can be confusing or you may prefer simultaneous readers. If so, keep track of your readers.

- Ask your readers specific questions that may include the following:
  - Is the layout reader friendly?
  - Could you understand all my directives? If not, identify where they are confusing.
  - Would different wording be clearer?
  - Is there any content in the caregiver handbook that is more appropriate for a lead caregiver handbook or key family handbook?
  - Would you suggest any other edits?

After working on this book for months and months, I was shocked when one of Rayna's caregivers who reviewed some pages made an edit about a list of necessities for a community bag to be ready at all times with items such as medical history papers, reusable shopping bags, water bottle . . . I had read that list hundreds of times throughout my writing and editing, yet she noticed something was missing and added Rayna's handicap placard to the list. Seriously? How can I be her mother and edit this handbook so many times yet leave out an important item like her handicap placard for parking? More eyes, deeper the vision.

Section E

Finished? Final Checks

In a sense, finishing a handbook is an oxymoron. Is a handbook ever finished? Short answer is yes. Long answer? Never. Yet finished enough for that moment. Life is not stagnant, and neither is your handbook. I try to measure my quest for perfection from an idiom my husband taught me, sage advice based on a phrase that is akin to the philosopher Voltaire, "Don't let perfection be the enemy of good."

Your goal is to place this handbook in your loved one's home and in the hands of her caregivers. Don't be hard on yourself; be gentle. Keep in mind you can edit at any moment. If you suddenly remember you forgot a directive or part of one or need to edit a directive, enter it in the appropriate place and reprint the page(s).

Readying the Handbook

First, choose your mode: print or electronic. I prefer printed. Although electronics are expedient and offer easier ways of editing, glitches such as power outages and charging issues can happen. In addition, I prefer that caregivers do not have access to Rayna's electronics.

If printing,

- continue to keep chapters in separate Word documents to make printing and assembly easier, as well as editing;
- use a colorful loose-leaf notebook with numbered dividers to match each chapter number.

Section F

Now What?

The answer is launch and keep current.

Launching Handbook

How you launch your handbook and who launches it depend on several factors:

- length of handbook
- number of caregivers
- time frame of how quickly you want information disseminated

Launching Handbook Options

- Train caregivers one-on-one or as a group. Zoom can be helpful.
- Leave handbook in household. Instruct caregivers to read entire book. Check with caregivers if they have any questions.
- Print out one chapter or section. Leave this chapter or section in caregiver mailbox if you chose mailboxes as part of your organizational system. Otherwise, leave chapter or section in the location you have designated for communication. If you choose this option, include a cover page with instructions to
  - read designated pages,
  - call key family with any questions,
  - initial cover page that materials have been read,
  - return pages to mailbox for other caregivers to complete this same assignment.
- Lead caregiver will remove pages from mailbox once all caregivers have initialed cover page.
- Newsletter

- Announce handbook is now in your loved one's home and specify selected training format.

You can combine options or create a different way to launch that suits you.

Keeping Handbook Current

My handbooks have been revised many times as Rayna's needs have changed and new ways to improve her life are identified. Yet I save old versions in case I want to revert to a former directive that I changed. Your handbook will evolve over time to ensure your loved one is taken care of now and in the future. Keep your handbook accurate and updated by amending information in appropriate chapter(s) and then printing pages to replace in handbook. Part 5, chapter 4, "KF Updating RS Information" has more details.

- Updates to handbook can be initiated by key family, suggestions from lead caregiver, caregiver(s), doctors, state officials, and any others involved in your loved one's care, including your loved one.
- Changes can include
    - new rules from housing management, if applicable;
    - new or revised contact information;
    - changes in medications;
    - new product for the "no" list;
    - system, thought effective, suddenly doesn't work;
    - changes in medical condition; and
    - changes from aging.

Each time you edit your handbook, remember to

- save it as a backup before you edit;
- rename version to be edited;
- continue to keep separate Word documents for each chapter for easier realignment;
- ensure that all caregivers are notified when there are handbook revisions; and
- print the page or pages with update(s), highlight that information, staple a message form that includes an initial strip at bottom of page, and put all this in caregiver mailbox.

Example of an Edit

When we changed location of backup cleaning supplies from under the sink to storage closet, message form looked like this:

> I have read the highlighted changes from chapter 1: "Introduction," section D about change in storage of backup cleaning supplies.
>
> Initial: _____ _____ _____ _____ _____ _____ _____

Once each caregiver signs the form, lead team caregiver removes this message form.

Note: Even if you have no amendments, periodically revert to launching options and/or a newsletter with a reminder to keep handbook fresh in caregivers' minds.

Part One Summary

Let's review!

- Don't assume! Be aware.
- Don't be hard on yourself! Be gentle.
- Don't use thesaurus words. Use everyday vocabulary.
- Don't get frustrated. Remember this is a labor of love in the truest sense.
- Don't relay crucial information verbally. Use "put and get" rule to *put* in writing and *get* initials.
- Do write a follow-up e-mail for a paper trail if you need to relay crucial information verbally.
- Do reach out for help in whatever capacity: family, friends, professionals, caregivers, lead caregivers, and loved one.
- Do put information in more than one chapter if needed.
- Do be detailed but not wordy; strong but not demanding.
- Do be clear. Be specific about what you are asking.
- Do use short sentences when possible.
- Do avoid essay style or free-form writing for communications. Do design forms requesting circling, checking off answers, etc., as much as possible.
- Do use bullet points to list directives clearly.
- Do organize your information according to subtopics.
- Do accept that perfection, while preferred, isn't always a reality. Aim for safe and happy.
- Do turn hiccups into opportunities to create positive changes.
- Do always remember this is *your* handbook to take care of *your* loved one.

Part Two

How to Create Handbooks for Lead Caregiver and Key Family

Ideally, your loved one's home should include one lead person and/or one key family member. However, your circumstances might not require this need and/or be feasible, so part 2 may not be applicable ever or for the moment, and you can now continue to the sample(s) starting in part 3.

When I hired privately, after working on a caregiver handbook for years, I concluded that some information only belonged in the hands of a trustworthy person in charge, so I sifted out certain directives and created a separate lead caregiver handbook. As I wrote this handbook, I again realized I included directives that really belonged in the hands of key family, so I repeated my filtering process, and a key family handbook was born!

Before we delve into how to create these handbooks, it's important to have a general overview of the caregiver(s) and key family roles. In addition, part 2 addresses the following:

- differences and similarities between caregivers and lead caregivers
- differences and similarities to creating a handbook for lead caregiver
- differences and similarities to creating a handbook for key family
- dual roles if one person serves in both capacities

Lead Caregiver

- No matter the title, lead caregiver, lead team member, lead staff, main staff, key team member . . . any person in charge is central to establish order and help prevent potential disorder.
- If possible, use someone who can be on site and even better if this person is part of your caregiving team.
- Even though key family engages a lead caregiver and has a handbook, he/she may still want involvement to some degree. Ideas:
  - Ask lead caregiver to share forms that caregivers complete documenting your loved one's care.

- Ask lead caregiver for weekly or monthly updates depending on your desire for frequency of communication.
- If key family is local,
    - spend a few minutes with lead caregiver, whether at random or designated times;
    - check physical condition of your loved one's home. Neat? Clean? Smells fresh? Items in appropriate location? Refrigerator stocked? Is your loved one clean and well groomed?
- If key family is not local,
    - set up a Zoom meeting with all caregivers, lead caregiver, and your loved one;
    - ask someone to stop by to assess living situation, and/or be willing to check in with your loved one should the need arise.

Possibilities for engaging a lead caregiver:

- Hire an agency that assigns a lead caregiver.
- Hire an agency that does not assign a lead caregiver.
    - Ask agency if amenable to you delegating one caregiver to be a lead caregiver. While not a requirement, the presence of a lead caregiver can be an asset to making the household run smoothly.
    - If not, and you still want to hire this agency, share thoughts about you engaging an outside person.
- Hire private caregivers; options are the following:
    - Appoint one caregiver to be a lead.
    - Engage an off-site lead caregiver, if on-site is not possible.

When engaging lead caregivers:

- Establish boundaries.
- Be clear in stating your needs and expectations of a lead caregiver.
- If using an agency, mesh your visions. They have certain requirements.
- Balance your position being involved with your loved one's life and day-to-day living with an agency's protocol. Make your goals clear but let them do their job.

In Rayna's household, our lead caregiver has several shifts, and she performs as caregiver and lead caregiver.

Possibilities for lead caregiver responsibilities:

- Act as a liaison between caregivers and agency and between caregivers and key family.
- Manage household.
  - Complete tasks assigned for lead caregiver only.
  - Communicate key family updates to caregivers.
  - Prepare house for weekend caregivers.
  - Manage key family-approved money for laundry, loved one's spending money, and incidentals.

Key Family

Although you engage caregivers, and possibly lead caregivers, there are many tasks that only a key family member prefers to complete. That is up to each family.

Key family can decide how much authority and information to allow a lead caregiver, such as the following:

- assigning and overseeing lead caregiver for certain tasks, such as preparing your loved one for travel
- coordinating deadlines for lead caregiver to assist in gathering supporting documents for key family to submit applications for town, state, and federal assistance, such as annual rebates and certifications
- authorizing access to select financial information
- authorizing access to select passwords

For several years before we secured our current agency, I acted as key family, hired privately, and I filled in as lead caregiver to the best of my ability. After dropping the lead caregiver role, I remained key family. Even if you retain this title, one day you might transfer your role to another family member or individual, so a key family handbook is essential.

Steps for creating a lead caregiver handbook and/or key family handbook have similarities to a caregiver handbook, yet some directives may be a new concept or need to be substituted. You do not have to repeat any directives from your caregiver handbook; simply refer to appropriate chapters.

Similarities

- mirroring mindset advice by eliminating "overwhelmed" and "daunting"
- writing styles
- needing household organized
- needing smoothly running communication systems
- gaining more confidence and experience, and catching your rhythm and style
- removing assumption from your vocabulary
  - You cannot assume. Assumptions and caregivers no more go together than assumptions in a handbook for lead caregiver and/or key family.
  - You cannot assume your expectations of your vision will be met.
  - You cannot assume key family, who one day may take over your reins, knows every task and responsibility.

Differences

- Substitute evaluating your loved one's needs with evaluating your goals for lead caregiver/key family.
- Set your expectations. What do you want their role(s) to look like?
- Evaluate how much responsibility they should or need to have.
- Decide what topics are similar, different, or need additional directives to what is included in the caregiver handbook.
- Determine if additional forms for lead caregiver and/or key family are necessary.

These preparatory steps will help you get organized to create an additional handbook(s).

Now let's look at some sample handbooks that demonstrate possibilities for you. These samples are composed of examples from a combination of the various editions of my handbooks, depending on the agencies I used as well as when I hired caregivers privately.

My samples might not cover every topic. Some may be universal, while others are very specific to Rayna whether because of her medical situation, results of hiccups, or are needed specifically for her lifestyle. My ideas of handling directives may not match yours, such as ways to handle your loved one if upset. These are only samples and suggestions. What works for Rayna may not work for your loved one. You might discover new topics, need additional directives, such as adding to the 911 emergency list or needing different directions for food preparation.

You also don't need to follow my systems. You might read a directive and think, "Wow, what a great idea," or "I would never do that," or "Some of that works." For example, you liked the organization I suggest for getting to and from laundry room, but your loved one might prefer her laundry be washed and dried in a different way. Your handbook for your loved one.

All set?

Part Three

Rayna's Team Member Handbook: Sample

CONTENTS

Author Note: This is where you would put the table of contents with corresponding page numbers for your handbook.

ORIENTATION

WELCOME! Your help and caring are most appreciated. Rayna loves life despite cognitive and physical challenges from a brain injury. She is bright, insightful, and inspiring.

- This sheet is a brief introduction to Rayna's team member handbook (binder on communication table behind living room recliner chairs). After reading, return sheet to basket.
- Please call Rayna by name—do not create nicknames. All references in handbooks except for chapter and section titles are referred to in shortened forms or initials: "RS" for Rayna, "TM" or "Team" for Team Member(s), "LTM" for Lead Team Member(s), "AGY" for Agency, "KF" for Key Family, and "AGY/KF" for Agency and/or Key Family.
- If you need help, call AGY/KF (names and numbers).

Text KF now with your name and cell number. To help RS remember, also make a TM contact card with your name and cell number and tape to left arm of RS recliner. When your shift ends, put your TM contact card in the basket on her recliner side table. Index cards and tape are in desk organizer on communication table behind recliners.

RS is at RISK of CHOKING and FALLING

- RS must wear the gait belt at all times except to shower and sleep, and you must always hold on to it. Walk a little behind RS (on her right side) and make sure she does not walk too fast. If you are not familiar with using a gait belt, you will find instructional videos on YouTube.
- Until you read handbook chapters 1 and 2, do not let RS exercise walk and do not leave RS alone in apartment.
- In addition, do not go out in the community unless scheduled. Call AGY if event arises.
- If RS must go out during your shift, take the community bag (bag with luggage tag under communication table), which contains the community booklet with chapter 5, "Community," and other instructions.

- Explain to RS you were asked to first read some of handbook and then you'd like to chat a little to get to know her.

- Read chapters 1 and 2 but stop reading if RS needs you. She is your number-one focus.

- Once you have read chapters 1 and 2, chat with RS unless she has fallen asleep or is talking on the phone, and then continue reading handbook unless meal preparation is required. Read chapter 4, "Daily Procedures," section D before any meal/snack preparation.

- Fill out message forms with information such as messages received or products used up, and put in turquoise mesh three-drawer organizer in communications center. Forms are on top of organizer.

- Listen carefully for any phone calls where RS might be giving out personal or credit card information. If you suspect this type of call, kindly take phone from RS and hang up. For more information, see chapter 4, "Daily Procedures," section F-2.

Thank you for coming in today!

HOW TO READ HANDBOOK

Some directives repeat on purpose because they apply to more than one topic.

Many pages end before the page is filled to make it easier to read a chart or list on one page. Chapter is not over until you see the end-of-chapter indication.

It is important to read the entire handbook as soon as possible. There are a lot of directives and details to know. Keep in mind the handbook is a resource to refer to as needed. For example, you are not expected to know all the steps and details on how to do RS laundry after one reading. But when it is your first time to do laundry, or if you need a reminder, simply go to the table of contents and look for the chapter and section(s) that specify laundry.

Chapter 1

Introduction

Orientation

How to Read Handbook

Section A: Rayna Communications

    A-1: Overview

Section B: Starting Shifts

Section C: Team Directions

    C-1: Agency Policies
    C-2: Team Rules
    C-3: Team Relations
    C-4: Team Meals
    C-5: If You Return for Another Shift

Section D: Apartment and Building

    D-1: Structure of Apartment and Building
    D-2: Apartment Organization
    D-3: Apartment Building Rules

Section E: Taking Care of Rayna

E-1: Overview

Section F: Daily Checklist Explained

Section G: Crisis Management

Section A: Rayna Communications

A-1: Overview

A message from Rayna:

> Thank you for coming in to take care of me and talk to me and get to know me. I want to get to know you, and I hope we have fun together!

RS is very intelligent and has many high-functioning capabilities; however, because of brain injury, she needs assistance in many areas. She often experiences slow comprehension and processing, forgetfulness, and difficulty with word retrieval, so frequent cueing is helpful.

Despite her challenges, RS should be actively involved in running her daily life as much as possible.

- Listen to RS—having her voice heard and being validated are very important.
- The most effective method to speak to or cue RS is to talk slowly with gentle tones while being patient and understanding.
- Get to know each other by asking RS about herself and sharing information about you.
  - Share favorite colors, food, movies, TV shows, likes and dislikes.
  - Share backgrounds: cultures, family histories, traditions, birthdays, and favorite recipes.
  - Never share inappropriate information, such as financial worries, intimate issues, or disturbing current events.
- RS might quickly forget what she wants to say or not grasp the word she wants.
  - Give her a chance to think of the word.
  - If this takes a long time or she gets frustrated, give her help such as asking her to describe what she's trying to say.
  - Suggest categories like "Was it about a food you want?" or "Were you wondering where we are going today?"
- If RS wants to talk to you at a moment when you are busy, ask for a key word. As soon as you finish your task, repeat key word to help her remember.
- Give RS only one task or one question or one choice at a time.
  - If you say, "Do this, this, and that," she may get confused and overwhelmed.
- Avoid asking "or" questions.
  - Example: "Do you like comedies or romance movies?" may cause a problem because by the time you say "romance," she might have forgotten the first choice of comedies.

Ask one question at a time: Ask, "Do you like comedies?" Let her answer and then ask, "Do you like romance stories?"

- Speak with positive words and tone. Never use derogatory language like "What is wrong with you?" or if she forgets, "I already told you," or "You already asked me that."
- We welcome suggestions.
  - If you have an idea to improve anything, including cleaning, cooking, or hygiene, KF wants to hear about it, so put a message form in LTM mailbox.
  - Do not share any suggestions with RS. It might not be something KF wants to pursue.
  - If you notice something seems broken or if you would like to suggest a brand of food different from what RS has in her home, don't mention it to RS, but leave a message for LTM.

Section B: Starting Shifts

- If you are on your way but running late, call RS home (number) to let current TM know you are on your way.
- Upon walking into RS home, you must *not* be on your phone.
- Greet RS.
- Throughout your shift, keep your charged cell phone on the right side of the dining table, which is referred to as dining table-TM side, unless you are leaving the apartment.
- Clock into AGY.
- Follow shift in/out checklist (on cover of Checklist binder on communication table).
- Check TM easel and TM mailbox.
- Tape your TM contact card to left arm of RS recliner.
- In case of any urgent messages, check cork/whiteboard (on wall above dining table) and red clipboard with medicine/fever form if on dining table-TM side.
- Review daily checklist (turquoise clipboard on dining table-TM side).
  - Daily checklist indicates tasks to be done. See section F at end of this chapter. Throughout your shift, initial tasks on daily checklist as they are completed.
- Review Checklist binder.
  - Review daily checklists since your last shift, or if you are new to RS care, review past three days.
  - Review RS Calendar (inside pocket of Checklist binder) for any events in the community (anything inside or outside of apartment building or anyone coming to RS home). Making sure RS is safe and ready to go out in the community is crucial. See chapter 5, "Community."
  - Review TM Calendar (inside pocket of Checklist binder) for weekly and monthly chores to be done that day. See chapter 4, "Daily Procedures," sections H and I.
- Daytime shift only: Determine if laundry needs to be done during your shift. If so, read chapter 4, "Daily Procedures," section C. Laundry is done on days RS showers and/or as needed for clothes and towels. LTM will alert you for days to wash blankets, sheets, and comforter.
- Attend to any tasks on daily checklist needed to be done immediately.

Section C: Team Directions

C-1: Agency Policies

- TM cannot leave until next TM arrives.
- TM may only leave RS alone in her apartment to go briefly to her car or apartment building dining room, laundry, offices, trash room, or mailbox.
- TM is not allowed to eat any of RS food, unless special occasion like birthdays or to taste a new recipe being prepared with RS.
  - Bring extra food in case next shift is called out or delayed.
- TM is not allowed to have any guests.
  - If someone is picking up TM, driver must wait outside building.

C-2: Team Rules

- TM must follow rules posted on pink card (wall 3) and also in chapter 2, "Medical and Safety," section B-1, before ever leaving RS alone.
- Smoking is not allowed in apartment or anywhere around RS.
- Do not change thermostat unless RS states she is cold or warm.
- Do not put personal belongings anywhere in RS home except in plastic bin by front door; however, you may leave your cell phone on dining table-TM side.
- Never use any of RS machines such as CPAP until you are trained by KF. Chapter 6, "Resources," has CPAP instructions to review.
- Never use any of RS electronics such as laptop or iPad without permission from KF.
- RS enjoys music.
  - Let RS choose the music.
  - Do not play music that is vulgar, about sex, with swears or violence in RS apartment, outside, or with her in your car.
- Engage RS in at least five positive activities daily. Details are at end of this chapter in section F.
- Do not use personal devices unless all tasks are completed and RS is sleeping or engaged in conversation with a friend visiting or on phone.
  - Check on her regularly, and as soon as she needs your attention, put away your personal devices.
- Making personal calls is not allowed. If you receive a call of an urgent matter or need to make a call that cannot wait until after shift, please be as brief as possible.

- Avoid upsetting RS. Try not to use words around her like "emergency" or imply something is seriously wrong with RS or someone else.
- Text information to AGY about any medical issues you do not understand—never discuss near RS.

C-3: Team Relations

- If you have an issue with another TM,
    - do not argue or discuss an issue with that TM;
    - if TM starts to speak to you about the issue, politely say to call AGY;
    - call AGY for assistance once you have left RS apartment;
    - never allow RS to know there is an issue. Keep it between you and AGY, and do not discuss with KF. AGY will inform KF if necessary.
- Do not discuss potentially upsetting news near RS.
    - If this happens on your shift, see chapter 3, "Communications," section B for further information.

C-4: Team Meals

- Never use RS dishes, silverware, cups, glasses, or utensils for eating or drinking.
- If you forget to bring a plate, cup, or utensil, ask RS for a paper or plastic one (located in top cabinet to right of refrigerator).
- You may sit at dining table-TM side.

C-5: If You Return for Another Shift

- If your car is not available, inform AGY well in advance of your shift. If RS has an event out in the community that day, AGY will do their best to arrange for transportation or they might need to get a sub for the day to replace you.
- Do not wear medical uniforms.
- Do not come to shift in clothing that smells of smoke.
- If you smoke in your car, please spray it before transporting RS.

Section D: Apartment and Building

D-1: Structure of Apartment and Building

Structure of Apartment Building

Main office	Water dispenser (lobby)
Resident assistant office	Dining room
Mailboxes (lobby)	Laundry room
Community room	Restrooms (across from laundry room)
Library	Trash/recycle room (next to laundry room)

Structure of RS Apartment

Dining Table

- Left side of table is where RS eats.
- Right side of table (referred to as "dining table-TM side") is for TM to use for paperwork and to keep your cell phone.

Plastic Bin

- All TM belongings must be kept in large plastic bin, to left of the bathroom. This includes coat, boots, tote bag, and pocketbook, except cell phone, which should always be kept on dining table-TM side.

Three Closets

1. Linen/coat closet to left of front door (for RS coats only)
2. Bedroom closet
3. Storage closet, across from front door, containing
   - backup inventory;
   - cabinet with products basket on top as well as a crafts basket to put unfinished activities RS is working on and wants to complete later, such as a thank-you note, greeting card, or crafts project;
   - transport wheelchair;
   - steamer, broom, and microfiber wipes;
   - cleaning products;
   - basin;

- storage bags with TM blankets for overnight shifts; and
- luggage.

TV Cabinet (to left of dining table under the wall with TV)

- on top: printer and Lifeline 911 button charger
- inside: extra computer paper

Photos Cabinet (to left of TV Cabinet)

- Lifeline 911 communication box (on top)
- RS landline and cell phone chargers (on top)
- photos and greeting cards received (on top)
- games (inside)

Communication Table (behind recliners)

- See chapter 3, "Communications," section A-1 for explanations of all materials on communication table.

Living Room Wall Units and Carts

- All wall unit drawers are labeled.
- Cart on left is daily medication center.
  - pill container, pill cups, and eye treatment supplies on top
  - various medical supplies in drawers
- Cart on right is art/stationery supplies.

Communication Wall 1 (above dining table)

- RF cork/whiteboard for red flag (crucial) information
  - See chapter 3, "Communications," section B.

Communication Wall 2 (on side of living room wall unit above daily medication center)

- eye treatment instructions

Communication Wall 3 (to right of storage closet)

- apartment lanyard with laundry card, apartment door key FOB, apartment building key, and mailbox key
- wooden clipboard with laundry sign-out form
- emergency contacts, how to call 911, and other urgent information
- pink card with rules for briefly leaving RS alone

Laundry Supplies Area

- white three-shelved bookcase to left of bathroom door

Kitchen

- "File of Life" for EMT is on freezer door.
- Mesh basket with labels and markers for labeling food is on side of refrigerator. See chapter 4, "Daily Procedures," section D-4.
- Garbage disposal switch is under the sink counter.

Phones

- In addition to RS cell phone, she has two landline phones: one only for TM and one only for RS.
- RS landline and cell phone chargers are on photos cabinet.
- TM landline phone charger is on dining table-TM side.

D-2: Apartment Organization

- Do not change locations of things in RS apartment. Problems result when something is not in assigned place.
- Drawers and cabinets are labeled. Pay attention when you take something out of a drawer or cabinet and return to same place.
- Products/papers that are delivered or picked up (except medications) go to storage closet.
- Medications that are delivered or picked up, go on dining table-TM side.
- Put message form in LTM mailbox where you have placed delivered or picked up item(s).

D-3: Apartment Building Rules

- Do not leave shoes, boots, or any objects outside RS door.
- Parking
    - row 1: handicap parking—never park there.
    - rows 2 and 3: residents
    - row 4: visitors—where you park, by the fence
    - If row 4 is filled, you may park in row 3.
    - If row 3 is also filled, park in 2 and notify apartment office you have parked there (number).
    - If office is closed, park in parking lot across the street and call KF.
    - Never park your car blocking the ramp at the front door. See chapter 5, "Community," section B-5 regarding parking to get RS in and out of your car.

Section E: Taking Care of Rayna

E-1: Overview

- RS responds well to tenderness yet not being babied. Achieve this by using gentle tones and light touch, such as an occasional squeeze on her shoulder or tap on her arm.
- Engage in conversation with RS throughout your shift.
- If RS is frightened, sad, frustrated, disappointed, or cries, let her have a moment and then try to change her mood with a question about something, some humor, a suggestion to say a gratitude, listen to music, or play a meditation on the Calm or Headspace app.
- Cueing RS is necessary for certain tasks, including brushing teeth and taking pills.
- For brushing teeth, stand next to RS to make sure she is stable—hold on to gait belt.
- See chapter 2, "Medical and Safety," section A for information about
  - RS pills
  - RS drinking water
  - RS dry eyes treatment
- After reading chapter 2, "Medical and Safety," take RS for an exercise walk. Walk routes are detailed in Exercise binder on communication table.
- For your first shift, walk inside apartment only. RS uses her cane and make sure she has on her ankle brace, compression stockings, arm brace, and gait belt.
- Remind RS to keep the cane to her side and not in front of her.
  - Window to stove is one lap. Goal is to walk five laps, if possible.
  - If she seems unsteady or very tired,
    - skip exercise walk;
    - try to do chair exercises listed in Exercise binder;
    - continue to reposition (see chapter 2, "Medical and Safety, section B-2); and
    - use transport wheelchair for outside fresh air when weather is good.
- For RS meals, read chapter 4, "Daily Procedures," section D before preparing any meals/snacks.
- For information on protecting privacy and credit cards, see chapter 4, "Daily Procedures," section F-2.
- If next shift calls out or is late, review chapter 4, "Daily Procedures," section G, as well as sections H or I, depending on whether you are covering a daytime or overnight shift.
- Before you leave, review shift in/out checklist (on cover of Checklist binder) to ensure you have completed all exit tasks.

Section F: Daily Checklist Explained

- Daily checklist indicates tasks for the day.
- There is one checklist per day for all TM to use.
- Each TM initials when she completes a task; some require circling as well.
- Do not initial or circle any task that you did not complete.
- Each shift picks up where last shift left off until daily tasks are all completed.
- Some tasks need to be done at certain times, as indicated on daily checklist.
- Other tasks, such as positive activities and PT/OT (physical or occupational therapy) exercises, may be done at any time.
- Some tasks, such as showering, are every other day, so make sure to check previous day's daily checklist to know if any of those tasks should be done on your shift, and if not, write "N/A" (not applicable) on daily checklist.
- Explanations or chapters to find explanations are listed below in alphabetical order.

Apartment chores: see lists in chapter 4, "Daily Procedures."

- **Section H** for 9:30 a.m.–9:30 p.m. chores
- **Section I** for 9:30 p.m.–9:30 a.m. chores

Ankle brace: stored inside shoes on bedroom back wall

Arm brace: stored in bedroom on top of tall bureau

Bedtime essentials: stored in nightstand

- mouth guard—in case marked "Mouth Guard"
- earplugs—in small, clear jar with green cover

Brush hair a.m.: see chapter 4, "Daily Procedures," section B-3.

- Have RS choose if she'd like her hair loose, put up in elastics, ribbons, and/or braided.

Brush hair p.m.: see chapter 4, "Daily Procedures," section B-3.

- If applicable, take out elastics, ribbons and/or braids, brush hair, and leave loose.

Brush teeth a.m. and p.m.: hold gait belt.

Charge cell phone: charger is on photos cabinet.

Clean ankle brace: after taking off ankle brace in evening, clean with alcohol wipe.

Clean eyeglasses: see chapter 4, "Daily Procedures," section B-4.

Community ready: see chapter 5, "Community," section A.

Compression stockings: stored in right top drawer of bedroom multicolored bureau

CPAP a.m.: see CPAP directions for cleaning in chapter 6, "Resources."

CPAP p.m.: fill water well with distilled water.

- It is crucial to use only distilled water (jug is on bottom shelf of bedroom beige wall unit).
- Be careful when filling water well to stop at maximum line.

Eye treatment: see chapter 6, "Resources" (also taped to side of left wall unit).

Gait belt: see chapter 2, "Medical and Safety," section B-2.

Laundry: see chapter 4, "Daily Procedures," section C.

Meals planned for the day: see chapter 4, "Daily Procedures," section D.

Mouth guard soak: see chapter 4, "Daily Procedures," section B-4.

Outside: ten plus minutes of fresh air (weather permitting)

- See chapter 2, "Medical and Safety," sections B-2 and B-5.

Pills a.m. and p.m.: see chapter 2, "Medical and Safety," section A.

Positive activities: can be done at any time

- There are five categories of activities:
  1. Say a gratitude.
  2. Play music (ask Alexa)—RS enjoys '60s, '70s, '80s music and show tunes.
  3. Choose Headspace or Calm (on YouTube app, TV, or RS phone).

4. Choose Ted Talks or Lumosity (on YouTube app, TV, or RS phone).

5. Choose game or crafts or cooking.

- Every day have RS choose at least one activity from each category.
- Once an activity is completed, circle on daily checklist.
- Encourage RS to vary activities.
  - If you see a lot of Ted Talks, suggest Lumosity.
  - If you see a lot of crafts, suggest playing a game, etc.

Prescription mouthwash: once a week after brushing teeth. (We chose Wednesday.)

- Use prescription mouthwash on bathroom shelf.
- Follow directions on label.

PT/OT exercises: see Exercise binder.

- PT/OT exercises are done once each day unless RS had session with PT/OT.

Reposition: see chapter 2, "Medical and Safety," section B-2.

Shower/Sponge bath: see chapter 4, "Daily Procedures," section B-1.

Sit-to-stand exercises: see Exercise binder.

Skin care: see chapter 4, "Daily Procedures," section B-2.

TheraTears: stored in daily medication center—one drop in each eye every two hours.

Walk routes: see Exercise binder.

Water cues and bottles: see chapter 4, "Daily Procedures," section D-2.

Wearing second-day clothes: see chapter 4, "Daily Procedures," section C-1.

Section G: Crisis Management

For all crisis events, call AGY/KF for advice to handle situation(s). Contacts are on wall 3 (to right of storage closet).

Crisis Definition

- RS-specific news, such as death in family or of a friend or if someone is diagnosed with a serious illness
- Crisis examples include natural disaster, pandemic, shooting in the area, etc.

Crisis Procedures

- Do not put on any news stations. If RS is watching a show and news comes on, quickly block the TV and distract her, such as ask a question about a meal or about trying a new recipe. Then as her show returns, you can stop the distraction.
- If you think you can't give her attention because you are at the stove or running to the laundry room, have her watch taped shows or Netflix.
- For any crisis, keep RS upbeat and happy, and do not bring up the crisis.
- If RS brings up the subject and/or asks a question, answer her honestly and directly. Do not offer more information than needed.
- Always add positive comments.
- Comfort her by gently squeezing her shoulder or lightly patting her arm.
- In addition to talking to RS,
  - play meditation on her phone or iPad (Calm or Headspace);
  - play music, sing, or play a game.
- Any threat to safety outside of the apartment, do not leave. Shut shades and stay away from the windows and door.
- Fill out a red flag (RF) corkboard form-back side for notes about RS emotional state. See chapter 3, "Communications," section B.
- For all crisis, contact KF.

END OF TM CHAPTER 1

Chapter 2

Medical and Safety

Section A: Medical Overview

RS was born with a genetic disorder and had a bleed in her brain at the age of three. She is very positive, loves life, and has a great sense of humor, despite the following challenges:

- weakness on her right side
- fall risk
- cognitive skills, such as memory problems, word retrieval, and slow word processing
- sleep apnea

Additional Medical Overview

- wears arm brace, ankle brace, and compression stockings per schedule on daily checklist
- wears gait belt
- wears medical alert bracelet
- wears a Lifeline 911 button
- takes pills twice a day, morning and evening—none are life-dependent medications.
  - Pill container is filled monthly by RS with KF supervision. If you encounter any problems, contact AGY/KF. Do not change any pills in pill container.
  - To take pills,
    - hold pill container so RS can open appropriate day, morning or evening;
    - have her put pills in a little medicine cup found in daily medication center or in kitchen drying rack;
    - cue her to take pills with water and watch her take the pills. You cannot place medicine cup next to RS, walk away, and assume she will take her pills; she could forget in that minute.
- RS must drink water throughout the day to avoid dehydration. She does not always remember to drink. You must remind her to drink water. On daily checklist schedule, circle number whenever she finishes a bottle.
- RS has dry eye syndrome and needs daily eye treatments:
  - Morning and evening treatments are detailed in chapter 6, "Resources."
  - Also, put in TheraTears eye drops every two hours and circle on daily checklist. (KF has set up Alexa with reminders.)
- Always check RS for any possible swelling.
- Updated medical history is always in community bag.
- For a full list of RS medication allergies and intolerances, see chapter 6, "Resources."

A-1: Contacts/Communication Chart

CONTACTS

Author note: This page is where you list all important contacts, such as

Apartment office/maintenance (if closed, ask for on-call person)
Resident assistant
Lifeline company
Primary care physician
Agency
Family list:

Key Family

List all others to contact in the order you want to be called if key family not available.

COMMUNICATION CHART

	SITUATION	ACTION	#1 Contact	#2 Contact
Emergency	For medical emergencies, see list on wall 3. (List is also in chapter 6, "Resources.") Any electrical issue, fire, flooding, or intruder in apartment	Call	911	
Urgent	See list of urgent situations on wall 3. (List is also in chapter 6, "Resources.")	Call	AGY	KF
Urgent	Any water leak, heat issue, or repairs needed	Call	Apt. office	KF
Urgent	Problem with Lifeline 911 button or charger	Call	Lifeline company	KF
Urgent	Locked out	Call	Apt. office	KF
Urgent	Smoke detector malfunction	Call	Apt. office	KF
Not Urgent	An issue with another TM (never discuss in front of RS)	Call	AGY	

Section B: Safety

B-1: General Safety Rules

- When RS sits in recliner, make sure she doesn't slouch. Cue her to sit as she was taught by her PT. See Exercise binder.
- When leaving RS apartment, never unlock the door. Always take apartment lanyard with you.
- During thunder or lightning storm, never let RS shower or talk on house phone.
  - Make sure cell phones are charged.
- Always shut off stove, oven, and toaster oven after use.
- Never leave any dish towels near the stove.
- Lifeline communication box is located on photos cabinet under the TV and must always be plugged in. See chapter 6, "Resources," for instructions.
- Only give RS medications on current medication list. See chapter 6, "Resources." Call KF for approval before giving any other medication to RS.
- Never leave things in RS pathways.
  - Anywhere RS might walk must be unobstructed to reduce the potential of tripping.
  - Make sure drawers and doors are closed.
  - Make sure brooms and vacuum cleaner are in storage closet.
  - Your personal belongings must be in plastic bin by front door, except for your cell phone, which must always be charged and on dining table-TM side.
- Rules for briefly leaving RS alone are at the end of this section.
  - Choose location card for your destination (index cards that say "laundry room" or "mailbox" etc., to leave with RS in case she forgets where you said you are going).
    - Location cards are in basket on RS recliner side table.
    - Tape is in desk utensil basket on communication table.
  - Tell RS where you are going and show her as you tape location card to left armrest of her recliner.
  - Upon return, remove location card from recliner and return to side table basket.

LEAVING RS ALONE—SAFETY RULES

CRUCIAL RULES WHEN LEAVING RS ALONE IN HER APARTMENT

- AGY rules mandate that you are not allowed to leave RS alone in her apartment, except to briefly go to your car or to apartment building dining room, laundry, offices, trash room, or mailbox.
- Rules for leaving RS are listed below and posted on pink card next to apartment lanyard on wall 3 to right of storage closet. You must read and follow these rules.

RULES FOR LEAVING RS ALONE

- RS is not sleeping in her bed.
- RS is in her recliner in living room and *awake.*
- RS has gone to the bathroom within the past thirty minutes.
- RS is not eating.
- RS is wearing her shoes and brace.
- You have told RS where you are going and taped location card on her recliner armrest.
- You have your cell phone, charged, and turned on in case RS needs to call you or you need to make a call for help to any of the following contacts (make sure you have these contacts saved in your phone):
  - RS H: (number) C: (number)
  - Agency: (name and number)
  - Key family: (name and number)
  - Apartment building office: (number)
- RS has her keys, two phones (home and cell), and water bottle next to her.
  - Never take RS keys with you. They must always stay in her recliner side table basket.
- You take apartment lanyard (wall 3 to right of storage closet).
- Never unlock door when leaving apartment—use apartment FOB to get into apartment. FOB directions are in chapter 6, "Resources."
- Hang up apartment lanyard upon return to apartment.
- Return location card to recliner side table basket.

B-2: Fall Risk

Although RS doesn't fall often, all TM must know how to try to avoid a fall as well as what to do if RS falls. (See wall 3). These fall-risk rules also apply to bed safety and outside safety in sections B-3 and B-5 in this chapter.

- Never let RS get up from sitting (chairs, bed, or toilet) without cautious supervision.
- RS feet fall asleep if she sits too long. She could fall getting up, so always be on alert. Tell her to shake her legs before standing, even if she says her feet don't feel asleep.
- RS must wear gait belt from the time she gets up until bedtime.
- In addition to gait belt, RS must use her cane whenever walking.
  - Hold gait belt using an underhanded grip with your palm toward you and firmly grasp the loop on the back of gait belt.
  - If RS loses balance, steady her with gait belt and help to regain balance.
  - Remind RS to keep the cane to her side and not in front of her.
- When she stands, make sure she is steady on her feet before walking.
- Walk a little behind RS (on her right side) and match her pace.
  - Remind her of safety walking procedures before she stands and while she is walking.
  - Remind RS to take her time when walking because she tends to walk too fast.
  - When standing or walking, cue her to stand straight, raise head, and put shoulders back, as leaning forward could cause her to fall.
  - Repeat: "Head up, shoulders back, look where you are going, no hunching over. Good job!"
- RS must reposition at least every two hours between her recliner with her feet up and a different chair with feet down.
- Cue her when moving from sitting to standing; see Exercise binder on communication table.

B-3: Bed Safety

- Never let RS get in or out of bed by herself.
- Raise or lower RS bed for her to get in or out.
  - RS will guide you how high to raise and lower her bed.
- Make sure she's not on edge of bed; otherwise, she could slip off and fall.
- Help RS put on CPAP.
- Whenever she wakes up, whether in the middle of the night or in the morning, before she stands, take off her CPAP and have her shake her legs in case they fell asleep.
- RS sleeps barefoot, but if she gets up to use the bathroom during the night, she must wear gripper socks (socks with ridges on the bottom).
- To help support RS, always try to put on gait belt before RS gets out of bed. If not possible, hold back of pants waist, and put on gait belt as soon as you can.
- See Exercise binder for sitting-to-standing techniques to get off bed.

- If it's not wake-up time and RS is returning to bed, once she is safely back in bed, help her put CPAP on. See chapter 6, "Resources."
- In bed, if RS complains about being uncomfortable, raise or lower bed and/or have her reposition her body.
- In an emergency, such as fire alarm, help RS remove CPAP, and use transport wheelchair.

B-4: Exercises

- Exercises are detailed in Exercise binder:
  - PT/OT exercises
  - Bed exercises
  - Chair exercises
  - Repositioning
  - Walk routes
  - Sitting to standing

B-5: Outside Safety

- When leaving apartment building, take apartment lanyard and your charged cell phone as well as either the medication pouch from community bag or entire community bag.
  - Bring medication pouch if taking a short walk or sitting outside the apartment building. Be sure to restock medication pouch with any Tylenol and/or Lactaid used and put back in community bag once you return to apartment.
  - Bring entire community bag if going beyond apartment building. See chapter 5, "Community."
- Hold on to gait belt when walking or use transport wheelchair.
- In addition to general walking rules listed above in section B-2 in this chapter:
  - Watch pavement and make sure surface is clear and even.
  - Never let RS walk on cobblestone, grass, sand, snow, ice, leaves, twigs, stones, or other objects or on wet pavement because she could fall.
  - Be careful of curbstones or even slight incline in sidewalk, either going up or down, which could cause RS to lose her balance.

B-6: Medical Safety

- Call AGY if you notice a medication or health issue out of the ordinary or that seems concerning to you.
- Only give RS medicine in wall unit pill container, pocketbook, or approved by KF.
- Never give RS any of your own medicine, even your own Tylenol.
- Never take any of RS medicine for yourself, even Tylenol.

B-7: Emotional Safety

How to keep RS emotionally safe when she is upset or scared:

- Acknowledge the issue even if you think it is not a reason to be upset.
- Never say, "You shouldn't be upset about that." Let her know you understand she is upset.
- If she cries, never say, "Don't cry." Give her a few minutes to cry, and then try to distract her.
- Speak slowly and gently but don't baby her.
- Ask RS what is bothering her.
- Suggest listening to her Headspace or Calm app.
- Play music—use Alexa.
- Always give RS a reason to be positive. Ask her to think of a gratitude.
  - For example, regarding the coronavirus pandemic, if she acts or says she is scared about getting the virus, assure her that TM are following all safety precautions and everyone is working hard to keep her safe.
- Suggest calling family or friend.

Call KF if RS exhibits unusual behavior, such as crying and unable to give a reason.

Section C: Emergency

Medical Emergency

List of symptoms and situations to Call 911 for medical emergency is posted on wall 3. List is also in chapter 6, "Resources."

How to Call 911

- Dial 911 using closest phone.
  - Alternative is to press RS Lifeline 911 button around her neck. Responder will answer through speaker in Lifeline 911 communication box.
- Provide RS address and phone number(s), RS cell, your cell.
- Remember to say, "Rayna has a brain injury."

If RS Goes to Emergency Room

- Once paramedics leave for ER, you will drive to ER.
- Bring community bag (under communication table with luggage tag).
- Take apartment lanyard so you can get back into apartment.
- Text AGY/KF to let them know you are going to ER. KF might be able to meet you there.

After 911 Emergency or Upon Returning from ER

- Contact AGY/KF (if KF did not meet you there) to let them know RS is home and follow AGY procedures.
- See chapter 5, "Community," section C, to determine items to leave, replace, or remove from community bag.

Nonmedical Emergency

- Sometimes it may be necessary to call 911 even if you have a nonmedical emergency, such as flooding. These emergencies might require immediate vacating.
- List of situations to Call 911 for nonmedical emergency is posted on wall 3. List is also in chapter 6, "Resources."

Section D: When Rayna Is Sick

- If RS is sick or shows any symptoms of getting sick, refer to wall 3 for list of symptoms that warrant a 911 call. List also in chapter 6, "Resources."
  - Take temperature and refer to wall 3 to establish if it is an emergency or nonemergency medical situation.
  - Thermometer is in left wall unit in second drawer labeled "RS Sick."
  - If you accidentally touch her forehead with the thermometer, clean it with an alcohol wipe.
- If 911 not necessary, refer to non-911 symptoms in chapter 6, "Resources." Then call AGY/KF, who may advise you to call her doctor or go to walk-in clinic.
- All contact numbers are in this chapter, section A-1, as well as in chapter 6, "Resources," and also posted on wall 3.
- If you are unable to reach someone, go to walk-in clinic.
  - name, address, number
- Continue to monitor RS and refer to nonemergency symptoms list to ensure that her symptom(s) do not escalate to a 911 situation.
- You are never allowed to leave RS alone when she is sick.
- If sheets, towels, or clothes are soiled, put in a plastic bag. Contact KF to get assistance for doing laundry.
- If you need food or medicine, contact KF.
- Never give medicine without permission from KF.
- Make sure RS is drinking extra liquids.
- When RS has a cold or flu, she likes to eat/drink
  - chicken noodle soup,
  - popsicles,
  - sorbet,
  - apple sauce, and/or
  - tea with honey.
- When RS has a stomachache or a stomach bug, she likes to eat/drink
  - ginger ale stirred to remove bubbles,
  - saltines with unsalted tops, and/or
  - tea with honey.

END OF TM CHAPTER 2

Chapter 3

Communications

Section A: Communications Overview

- RS household developed communication systems to provide consistent care for RS.
- Written communications are necessary to reduce misunderstandings and omission of important details.
- All communications must be initialed.
- Many communications must be initialed and left where found, unless you were directed to leave them elsewhere.
- Print clearly, even if only initialing.
- Use pencil only for calendar and pen for all other communications.

A-1: Locations

The long table behind recliners, right side of RS dining table, and several walls throughout apartment are used for communications.

- Long table is referred to as "communication table."
- Right side of dining table is referred to as "dining table-TM side."

Communication Table

- **Orientation basket**
  - Orientation sheet
- **Binders**
  - Checklist binder
  - Food/Recipe binder
  - Exercise binder
  - TM handbook binder
- **Mailboxes** (turquoise mesh three-drawer organizer with blank message forms on top)
  - **LTM mailbox** for messages and paperwork for LTM, such as lab slips, receipts, invitations, and flyers
  - **TM mailbox** for messages and communications from LTM to all TM or to a particular TM
  - **KF mailbox** for messages, papers, or items for KF
- **Contacts/passwords book** with names, addresses, phone numbers, and KF-approved passwords. If you encounter any information, such as new contact name, change of

address, change in password, phone number, office location closed or new one opened, put message form in LTM mailbox with new information.

- **Desk organizer** with pens, pencils, tape, scissors, notepads, location and contact cards
- **Communication basket**—black mesh basket containing
  - Red clipboard with RS medicine/fever form,
  - Forms folder for extra forms. For master forms, see chapter 6, "Resources."
- **Community bag** (luggage tagged bag under communication table). See chapter 5, "Community."

Dining Table-TM Side

- **Daily checklists** (on turquoise clipboard)
- **Team notes** (on TM easel)
- **Medicine/fever form** (on red clipboard)

Walls 1, 2, and 3: see chapter 1, "Introduction," section D-1.

Section B: Written Communications

A chart to guide you when to use message forms, team notes, or RF corkboard forms is at the end of this chapter.

Daily Checklist: see chapter 1, "Introduction," section F, for an explanation of daily tasks. Checklist is also in chapter 6, "Resources."

Checklist Binder

- Shift in/out checklist on front cover
- Past days' daily checklists
- RS Calendar in front pocket, unless in community bag
- TM Calendar in front pocket

Team Notes (on TM easel)

- Blank team notes are in TM easel front yellow pocket.
- If reading a team note, initial each team note once read.
- If writing a team note, address the information as needed and initial.
- When note is no longer needed to be posted, LTM removes it.

Message Form to LTM

- Put message forms in LTM mailbox.
- For urgent messages, text or call AGY/KF and complete RF (red flag) corkboard form—see section below for more RF information.
- At the end of this chapter, you will find a chart to guide you whether your message is red flag, urgent, or nonurgent.
- When in doubt about urgency of message, write LTM message form and call AGY/KF.

RS Calendar Entries

- Only use pencil when writing in calendar.
- Always put question mark next to event if pending.
- Always print clearly—no cursive handwriting.
- Write straight across and not at an angle.
- Do not fill up the entire date in case other events need to be entered.

- Whenever you make a calendar entry, put message form in LTM mailbox with all details:
  - name
  - phone number
  - date of event
  - address of event
  - scheduling conflict if there is one
  - gift or food donation needed
  - dress code in case RS needs to purchase outfit

Laundry Sign-Out Form

- On wooden clipboard on wall 3 (to right of storage closet)
- See chapter 4, "Daily Procedures," section C-3.

Red Flag Communications

Red flag (RF) is crucial information to be communicated immediately to all TM and KF.

- Although RF situations are infrequent, everyone must know about RF corkboard forms, whiteboard messages, and medicine/fever forms to convey relevant information. See RF examples at end of this chapter.
- Whenever TM has an RF situation happen on shift, call AGY and KF and follow these steps:
  - Fill out RF corkboard form, tack on cork/whiteboard and send a text to all TM.
  - If the RF on your shift involves RS becoming sick, see chapter 2, "Medical and Safety," section D.
  - Activate medicine/fever form if applicable. (Forms folder in communication basket).

RF Corkboard Forms

- RF corkboard forms are two-sided on pink paper in Forms folder in communication basket.
- **Front** is for information relating to medical issues such as RS is sick, new diagnosis, wound care needs, or new medication.
- **Back** is additional medical information if needed, as well as to alert TM and explain if RS is upset. Examples of emotional red flags are at end of this chapter.

- After filling out RF corkboard form, tack on corkboard side of cork/whiteboard (located on wall 1).
  - When LTM returns to shift, she will remove RF corkboard form and communicate any updates about RF situation on whiteboard side of cork/whiteboard.
  - Corkboard side is only used for TM to post RF corkboard forms.
  - Whiteboard side is only used for LTM to update RF situations.
  - At the beginning of every shift, check RS cork/whiteboard.

Medicine/Fever Form

- If at start of shift, you see an RF corkboard form or whiteboard message that RS is sick and medicine/fever form is already activated, continue to fill out that medicine/fever form.
- If during your shift, RS gets sick and/or starts a medicine, such as an antibiotic or Tylenol, start a medicine/fever form and indicate on RF corkboard form, and contact KF.
  - Put medicine/fever form on red clipboard (in communication basket) and leave on dining table-TM side.
  - Medicine/fever form stays on dining table-TM side until illness is over.

Examples of Message Forms, Team Notes, and RF Corkboard Form Communications

Message Form to LTM	Team Notes	RF Corkboard Form (front)	RF Corkboard Form (back)
Something needs to be ordered or picked up—also text KF.	TM didn't complete a task on daily checklist and reason why.	New crucial information or changes in medical information	Any additional information from front of corkboard form
Call from a doctor with information that is not time-sensitive for a response the same day	RS feet hurt from a lot of walking, and she may need transfer wheelchair in apartment.	RS is ill and you start medicine/fever form.	Odd behavior or comment beyond the ordinary
RS wants to buy tickets for a new show coming to the area.	TM took out frozen food and didn't have a chance to cook it.	Change of medicine that starts that day	RS receives bad news about someone
RS gets an invitation and wants to bring a gift and/or food item to event, and/or buy a new outfit.	Friend visiting in morning—finish birthday card if not tired.	New medical directives such as wound care to do on shift	RS hears of a crisis event
RS expresses she wants something in a store or from a TV ad.	Something is broken, and TM called maintenance and notified LTM.		RS is worried about an upcoming medical test.
Any medical information or upcoming test (attach paperwork)	RS wants to call someone on birthday or anniversary.		RS is worried about a family or friend.
RS liked or didn't like a new food or new product.	Unfinished craft project or greeting card, thank-you note		RS is worried or frightened in general.
New PT/OT exercises			

END OF TM CHAPTER 3

Chapter 4

Daily Procedures

Section A: Introduction to All Team Procedures

Section B: Hygiene

    B-1: Showering/Sponge Bath
    B-2: Skin Care
    B-3: Brushing Hair
    B-4: Cleaning Accessories

Section C: Clothing and Laundry

    C-1: Clothing
    C-2: Laundry Overview
    C-3: Preparing for Laundry Room
    C-4: Laundry Room
    C-5: Dryers and Finishing Laundry

Section D: Food and Kitchen

    D-1: Overview
    D-2: Food and Drink
    D-3: Meals and Snacks
    D-4: Kitchen

Section E: Physical Activity

Section F: Phone Calls

Section A: Introduction to All Team Procedures

In the pages that follow, you will find detailed descriptions of all procedures for RS day-to-day needs. Please read this entire chapter for a solid global understanding and to be prepared to cover another shift, if needed.

Section B: Hygiene

B-1: Showering/Sponge Bath

- RS usually showers every other day unless she gets sweaty or just wants to shower. On alternate days, she gets a sponge bath.
- Before sponge bath,
  - Close lid to toilet seat and have RS sit,
  - Lay down bathroom floor rug, and
  - Fill basin (from storage closet) with warm water.
- After sponge bath,
  - Hang bathroom floor rug over handicap bar to prevent mold,
  - After RS is dressed, empty the basin, dry it, and clean with disinfectant wipe, and
  - Return to storage closet.
- Before shower,
  - Lay down shower mat and bathroom floor rug and
  - Place towel in warmer twenty minutes before shower and plug in warmer.
- After shower,
  - Make sure hair is pulled back so not in eyes so she can safely transfer out of shower,
  - Close lid to toilet seat and have RS sit to dry off,
  - Make sure feet are dry and help RS dry between her toes,
  - Hang bathroom floor rug over handicap bar to prevent mold,
  - Hang shower mat over shower rod to prevent mold,
  - Unplug towel warmer,
  - Make sure cord is tucked away to avoid tripping, and
  - Always keep warmer unplugged when not in use.
- Circle "sponge bath" or "shower" on daily checklist.

B-2: Skin Care

If possible, when not going directly out in the community, allow a half hour for cream to dry before putting on compression stockings, slippers, and/or gripper socks. Compression stockings are stored in top-right drawer of bedroom multicolored bureau.

CeraVe Moisturizing Cream (located in living room in left wall unit, middle shelf)

- Once a day, apply CeraVe Moisturizing Cream to torso, arms, legs, and feet (soles, toes, and tops).
- Make sure RS feet and area between toes are dry before applying CeraVe Moisturizing Cream.

B-3: Brushing Hair

- Brush, comb, hair dryer, hair rake, and hair accessories are in left wall unit, middle shelf.
- Brush RS hair in the morning and as necessary during the day.
- Morning: Have RS choose if she'd like her hair loose, put up in elastics, ribbons, and/or braided.
- Evening: Remove any elastics, ribbons and/or braids, brush hair, and leave hair loose.
- Although brushes and combs are cleaned once a month, if you see that brush or comb has a lot of hair, use hair rake.

B-4: Cleaning Accessories

See TM calendar for schedule.

Ankle Brace/Arm Brace

- After taking off ankle brace in evening, clean with alcohol wipe (top drawer of medication cart).
- Arm brace is washed in mesh bag and air-dried. Directions below in section C.

Eyeglasses

- Use soft cloth in middle drawer of medication cart.
- Put cloth in laundry basket to wash in mesh bag with towels.

Gait Belt

- Hand wash and hang on shower rod to dry. (Use backup gait belt).

Mouth Guard Soak

- Return mouth guard to container.
- Pour in enough hydrogen peroxide to cover mouth guard.
- Soak for only thirty minutes—longer soaking could damage mouth guard.
- Rinse and dry mouth guard and container.
- Return container with mouth guard to nightstand.

Section C: Clothing and Laundry

C-1: Clothing

- RS dirty clothes (except for compression stockings) are put in tall laundry basket with wheels (to right of multicolored bureau).
- Put dirty compression stockings in colorful rattan basket next to laundry basket.
- When RS changes into nightgown/pjs,
  - check daily checklist if her clothes are second day, and if so, put in laundry;
  - if "second-day clothes" is not checked off on daily checklist and clothes are not soiled or sweaty, fold clothes and leave on multicolored bureau.
- When RS gets dressed in clothes found on multicolored bureau, check off "second-day clothes" on daily checklist so evening TM will know to put clothes in laundry basket.
- If RS is going out in the community for a social event, clothes are chosen day before and will be on hangers on closet doorknob.
- If weather changes or RS changes her mind what to wear, revise her outfit accordingly.

C-2: Laundry Overview

- Laundry is done
  - on shower days;
  - when needed for unexpected dirty laundry; and
  - for specific laundry, such as comforters, per TM Calendar.
- Laundry includes
  - clothes;
  - bedding, towels, bathroom rugs, eyeglass cloth; and
  - compression stockings, bras, and arm brace, which are all washed in a mesh bag and hung to dry. Mesh bag is under the compression stocking bin.

- All laundry baskets are to right of multicolored bureau.
  - Foldable white mesh basket is for *clean* clothes.
  - Tall basket on wheels is for *dirty* clothes.
- Laundry supplies are on three-shelf cabinet to left of bathroom door:
  - dryer sheets
  - laundry detergent
  - stain stick
- Laundry sign-out form and apartment lanyard are on wall 3 (to right of storage closet).

C-3: Preparing for Laundry Room

- Sign out laundry card on laundry sign-out form.
- Make a note of amount of money on card.
- Do not do laundry if there is less than five dollars on the laundry card and leave message form for LTM and call or text KF to refill card.
- Take apartment lanyard with laundry card.
- Remember to take all needed supplies:
  - dirty laundry cart
  - stain stick
  - laundry detergent
- Never leave RS alone without following rules on pink card on wall 3 (to right of storage closet).

C-4: Laundry Room

- Machine to refill money on laundry card is on left as you enter room.
- Insert laundry card and make sure amount matches amount on laundry sign-out form.
- If amounts don't match, write the amount machine says, and when you get back to RS apartment, put message form in LTM mailbox with both amounts.
- Separate clothes from sheets and towels, and separate dark clothes from light clothes.
- Put in items to be washed, then soap, followed by card.
  - Laundry card must be in slot in machine before you press start.
  - Do not throw away laundry detergent bottle or spray pump if used up. See section C-5 below.
- Wash clothes and mesh bag in cold water.
- Compression stockings are washed in white mesh bag along with bras (hook them) and arm brace.

- Wash towels, washcloths, and sheets in hot water.
- Note times: Washer takes forty minutes and dryer takes sixty minutes.
  - Return within forty minutes to move clothes to dryer or within sixty minutes to remove clothes from dryer.
  - Laundry room services entire building, and we do not want residents taking RS laundry out of washer or dryer.
- Before leaving laundry room, make sure you take apartment lanyard and have
  - stain stick;
  - laundry detergent bottle with sprayer (even if bottle is empty); and
  - dirty laundry cart, even if you need to put in additional washes.

C-5: Dryers and Finishing Laundry

Dryer

- Remember to take apartment lanyard.
- Take dryer sheets to laundry room.
- Never put the following items in dryer: bras, compression stockings, arm brace, sweaters, jeans, dresses, or jackets.
- When in doubt if something should go in dryer, leave out.
- Add one dryer sheet for each load in the dryer.

Finishing Laundry

- Use clean laundry mesh basket for carrying clean clothes.
- Hang apartment lanyard on hook.
- Write remaining amount of money on laundry card on laundry sign-out form and initial. If under ten dollars is left on laundry card, leave message form for LTM.
- Put compression stockings and bras on hangers and hang on closet door.
- Put arm brace on a towel and lay on top of bureau.
- Put empty mesh bag back under compression stocking bin.
- Fold jeans and sweaters over hangers and hang on shower rod.
- Hang any dresses and jackets with directions to air-dry on shower rod.
- Hang dry clothes in bedroom closet.
- Fold laundry and put away in designated drawers, bureaus, and linen closet.
  - If you do not know where items go, leave in mesh laundry basket and post a team note on TM easel asking next shift to put away.

- If you finish any laundry products,
  - put message form in LTM mailbox with information of what was used up,
  - never throw out detergent bottle spray pump, and
  - bring back to apartment and move spray pump to new detergent bottle. Replace spray pump when needed.
- Return laundry baskets to RS bedroom.

Section D: Food and Kitchen

D-1: Overview

- All shifts are responsible for meals, whether planning, preparing, or cleaning up.
  - When planning meals, check Food/Recipe binder (on communication table) to ensure variety of foods and involve RS in decisions about what she would like to eat.
- All shifts are responsible for keeping food calendar, writing what RS ate each meal.
- Keep opened food in original boxes. If need to clip packaging to keep product fresh, clips are in drawer to left of stove. Put packaging back in original box to know expiration date.
- If box damaged, put food in plastic bag and write expiration date on bag.
- Always use RS plates, bowls, and glasses when RS eats at home; however, when taking food out in the community, use paper products (in top cabinet to right of refrigerator).
- Keep RS company whenever she eats and sit near her. She occasionally falls asleep with food in her mouth and is at risk of choking, so give her your full attention. You are welcome to eat your meal with her, but keep your focus on her and do not work on other things while RS is eating.
- RS usually eats breakfast in her recliner and then has her eye treatment.
- Encourage RS to eat at dining table for lunch and/or dinner yet consider what she has been doing or is going to do later that day. If she is tired, let her eat at her recliner.
  - If she stays in her recliner to eat, use laptop desk (next to microwave), and sit across her in TM dining chair to keep her company.

D-2: Food and Drink

Hydration

- To avoid dehydration, RS must drink water throughout the day. See Food/Recipe binder.
- RS will not necessarily initiate drinking water—you must cue her.
- You must watch her and ensure that she drinks more than a little sip.
- When RS finishes a bottle, refill it and circle bottle number on daily checklist.
- After RS goes to bed, spill out any remaining water, wash empty bottle (using just a small drop of soap), rinse bottle thoroughly to remove all soap, and leave in drying rack.

D-3: Meals and Snacks

Meal Planning

- Food/Recipe binder on communication table is to keep track of RS food consumption and to follow directions to ensure she is eating a healthy variety of foods, such as getting greens and other vegetables with her meals.
- Always try to use leftovers before they spoil.
- Except for leftovers, avoid preparing same foods each day as much as possible.
- Before defrosting food from freezer, check Food/Recipe binder for foods she has eaten in past three days and try to vary meat, poultry, fish and vegetarian meals.
- Encourage her to vary snacks every day. Snack suggestions include fruit with peanut or almond butter, fruit with nuts, hummus and vegetables, or a treat of frozen yogurt (full list in chapter 6, "Resources").
- Encourage her to have a Shaklee smoothie (recipe in Food/Recipe binder). She can have one a day if she wants.
- Food Allergies and Intolerances. See wall 3 and chapter 6, "Resources."
- Product preferences, portions, and food guidelines are in chapter 6, "Resources."

Preparing

- Measuring is very important for meals and snacks. Portion guidelines are in chapter 6, "Resources."
- Always wash fruits and vegetables with fruit and vegetable spray kept next to sink, even if food is organic. Spray just a little and then rinse thoroughly.
- Always run cold water while using disposal.

- Follow recipes and/or methods RS has expressed for how she likes her food cooked. See Food/Recipe binder.
- Only cook/bake in roasting pans (with parchment paper) or glass or stainless-steel cookware.
- When RS eats a fruit snack, she should also eat a protein—for example,
  - fruit with nuts;
  - fruit with dairy, such as a slice of cheese or yogurt. When Rayna eats dairy, give her Lactaid chewable tablets. Follow instructions on bottle.
  - Lactaid tablets are in bottom drawer of medication cart.

D-4: Kitchen

Groceries

- Add to shopping list any products used up or getting low.
- Put away groceries as needed,
  - if LTM shopped for food yet didn't have time to put items away.
  - if groceries are delivered during your shift.
- Poultry, meat, or fish
  - Divide into portions to be frozen and put in freezer bags, and mark bags with contents and date.
- Produce
  - Break apart bunches of bananas and put in wire basket on top of refrigerator.
  - Put fruits in right drawer and vegetables in left drawer.
  - Move any vegetables or fruits found in wrong drawer.
  - Leave fruit that is not ripe on counter.
  - Check any fruit on counter that has ripened and put in refrigerator.

Products

- *Never* throw out or recycle used product containers until you put a message form in LTM mailbox with the product, brand, and flavor.
- Notify LTM if product running low.
- Notify LTM of changes in RS food preferences.
  - Put message form in LTM mailbox explaining if RS likes or dislikes a particular product or wants to try a different brand and/or flavor.

Labeling

- All cooked leftover or pre-cooked foods must *always* be labeled.
  - Write name of food, even if obvious, and date cooked.
  - Print clearly. Use number and day of month (i.e., March 22 would be 3/22).
  - Refrigerated leftovers must be used within two days or put in freezer.
- Never give unlabeled leftovers to RS. If unsure of date, send text to all TM asking date specific food was prepared. If food was made more than two days ago or if no one knows date, toss out item(s).
- Be aware of product expirations and foods that must be used within a certain date after opening.
  - Possible information on product: "Use within 7 days after opening" or "Use within 3 days after opening."
  - Label date when product is opened, and in parentheses, how many days good for, such as "10/22 (3)."

Freezer—when raw or cooked food is removed from freezer, add label with date removed:

- Put uncooked food package in a bowl or on a plate and defrost in refrigerator.
- Leave cooked food in container to defrost in refrigerator.
- Do not refreeze any defrosted food.
- Any raw piece of chicken/turkey, meat, or fish that was not cooked on day taken out of freezer must be cooked the next day.
  - If RS doesn't want to eat it that day, or the next day, label cooked food with date cooked and put in freezer.
- Any cooked dish defrosted must be eaten within two days.
- If you need next shift to cook a meal you planned to cook, write a team note and post on TM easel that food taken out of freezer needs to be cooked that day.

Cleaning Kitchen

- Each TM is responsible for daily cleaning. See chapter 6, "Resources."
- If you frequently notice the kitchen was not properly cleaned, put message form in LTM mailbox reporting this problem.

Section E: Physical Activity

- Before taking RS for any walks, see chapter 2, "Medical and Safety," section B.
- Details of exercise activities are in Exercise binder on communication table.
- When finished doing an exercise activity, mark on daily checklist.

Section F: Phone Calls

F-1: Overview

- TM is not to make or receive personal calls during shift.
  - If you receive a call of an urgent matter or need to make a call that cannot wait until after shift, please be as brief as possible.
  - Try not to use any words that might upset RS, whether directly to RS or that she might overhear.
  - If you need to leave your shift in an emergency, call AGY/KF for help.
- All phone communications for medical appointments and social events are handled by LTM, yet phone calls that need to be addressed may come in during your shift. See sections F-3 and F-4 in this chapter.
- RS has two portable landline phones and one cell phone.
  - TM landline charger is on dining table-TM side.
  - RS landline phone and cell phone chargers are on photos cabinet.
- TM is *only* to use TM phone whether answering, making calls on behalf of RS, or signing in or out with AGY. Never use RS cell phone or landline. If used by mistake, clean phone with a disinfectant wipe.
- If RS is sleeping or busy when cell phone rings, answer and take a message. When done, clean phone with a disinfectant wipe.
- If RS is sleeping or busy when landline phone rings, answer using TM phone, and take a message.
- Never leave RS in the shower to answer the phone—let phone ring. If you are expecting a return call such as from a doctor, take TM phone and RS cell phone into bathroom.
- If RS gets a call on your shift that something she ordered has arrived, text KF and put message form in LTM mailbox with relevant information.
- Other than social calls from family and friends, you must help RS with phone calls.
- When RS gets a call, if possible, stop whatever you are doing to listen and determine type of call—social, doctor's office, invitation, scam, or solicitation. (If RS sounds like she is trying to buy a product or give money, see next section for directions).

F-2: Protecting Privacy and Credit Cards

Protecting Privacy for all Personal Information and Credit Cards

- Never let RS give out her first and/or last name, address, home and/or cell phone, or social security number.
- RS credit card is kept in her wallet in the Community Bag.
- If she asks for the card, you are never allowed to get it for her without checking with KF.
  - If she wants it to order from an infomercial or to donate to a charity, have her give you all information.
  - If the need is to order something online, tell her to put it in the cart of the website.
  - Assure her all the information will be given to her KF to review and guide her. Never ask or remind RS about product or donation. Let KF talk to her and guide her.

Privacy from Unknown Callers

In addition to calls from known callers, such as doctors, companies, and associations, RS needs assistance with phone calls that might be scams, robotic calls, or solicitations for products and/or charity. TM have been cooking or in bedroom putting away laundry, and suddenly, RS is starting to give our personal information to an unknown caller or calling a telephone number she sees on TV. To protect RS privacy, follow these guidelines:

- If you are doing a chore, listen carefully to her talking on the phone to hear if she is trying to spend money.
- If you answer TM phone and call is solicitation or scam, do not respond. Hang up.
- If RS answers, get her to hang up. If RS starts to give any information, take over and either hang up or tell caller to give you all their information.
- If RS sounds like she is trying to buy a product or give money,
  - tell RS you will help her and talk to person on phone;
  - do not use RS phone; use only TM phone (on dining table-TM side); and
  - ask person about all product information and/or how to donate to charity;
- If RS gets upset, assure her that you will give information to KF;
- Put message form in KF mailbox with all information; and
- If you need to leave the apartment for laundry room, mailroom, etc., remind RS not to answer a call if she doesn't recognize the caller ID.

Protecting Privacy and Credit Cards from the Internet and Television Ads

- Supervise her e-mails and never let her respond to unknown e-mails asking for personal information.
- Avoid RS watching product-selling shows like QVC and HSN.
- Distract her to a different channel or turn off TV, watch a movie, or play a game.
- If she insists on watching, let her, and if she sees a product she wants, assure her you will give information to KF. Write all product information, price, and how to order on a message form and put in KF mailbox.

If you must leave RS alone briefly, to go to laundry room or dining room, or run to your car, ask RS to switch TV to Netflix or put on music until you return. Record TV show she is watching so she can resume watching show when you return.

F-3: Medical Appointments

- When phone call is to confirm a medical appointment, check RS Calendar and confirm.
- If doctor or medical facility calls to make or change appointment, ask caller to hold on or get name and number to call back. Immediately, call AGY/KF using your cell phone.
- Calls asking questions about appointments or to preregister should be referred to AGY/KF, who might advise to put message form in LTM mailbox with information.

F-4: Social Events

- All nonmedical events, whether casual, formal, or a meeting, are referred to as "social events." See chapter 5, "Community," section A.
- If invitation comes as a phone call,
  - help RS ask friend, relative, or organization for information about event and take notes;
  - check RS calendar, and if no conflict that day, she can accept the invitation; and
  - if RS has a conflict, have her tell caller she will try to reschedule and will call back. Leave message form for LTM with all information including if invitation was accepted or pending.
- If RS gets a call and wants to get together that day, confirm with AGY/KF, and if approved, help RS make the arrangements.
- If going out for a meal, ask friend/relative to pick a restaurant where it's easy to park and enter the building. Also, ensure seating has a movable table to facilitate RS getting in and out.

Section G: Bedtime and Wake-Up

This section is combined for day and overnight shifts because times for going to bed and for waking can overlap shifts.

Remember RS is at risk for falling. See chapter 2, "Medical and Safety," sections B-2 and B-3 for directions to help her get in and out of bed.

Bedtime

- Plug RS cell phone into charger on photos cabinet and return her landline to charger.
- Check RS Calendar to see if any events are planned for next day, and if so, remind RS of the event.
- Plan wake-up time per chart at end of this section, and write a team note about next morning's wake-up time and post on TM easel.
- RS sleeps barefoot.
- RS likes to be in bed by 10:00 p.m. or earlier if she seems tired.
- Before putting on bedtime essentials (ear plugs and mouth guard) and CPAP, TM should pull up a chair to RS bedside and visit with her.
- Help RS put on CPAP mask.
  - Instructions regarding CPAP machine are in chapter 6, "Resources."
- Make sure monitors in bedroom and living room are on and RS can be heard.
- If RS awakens during the night and when she gets up in the morning, see chapter 2, "Medical and Safety," sections B-2 and B-3.

While RS Is Asleep

- Even though monitors are on, do not wear earphones when listening to your electronic devices and keep on low volume.

Wake-Up Times

- Wake-up chart guides you for times to wake RS based on showering and/or when going out in the community.
- RS alternates shower days with sponge bath days unless she has an unusual situation, is sweaty, or just feels like a shower. Daily checklist indicates which day is shower or sponge bath.

WAKE-UP CHART

Calendar	Wake-up and Shower	Wake-up and Sponge Bath
Community before 1:00 p.m.	1.5 hour before leaving for event	1 hour before leaving for event
Community after 1:00 p.m. or No community for the day	8:00 a.m.–9:00 a.m.	8:00 a.m.–9:00 a.m.

Section H: Daytime Shift (9:30 a.m.–9:30 p.m.)

- For details on starting and ending shifts, see chapter 1, "Introduction," section B.
- Complete daily checklist throughout the shift.
- Follow chart in section G in this chapter.
- If RS is going out in the community, see chapter 5, "Community."
  - Getting ready for community is top priority, but if you are running late, tasks below with * may be skipped until you return.
- Brush teeth.
- *Shower/sponge bath.
- Apply creams—see section B-2 in this chapter.
- Get dressed.
- As close to 10:00 a.m. as possible, depending on when RS awakens, put on compression stockings, ankle brace, shoes, and arm brace.
- Compression stockings, ankle brace, and arm brace are to be worn according to schedule on daily checklist (see chapter 6, "Resources").
- Do eye treatment.
  - RS may eat breakfast during the waiting times between eye treatment drops (unless going for a test that requires fasting).
- Pills: Cue RS and watch that she takes pills.
  - RS takes morning pills with or immediately after breakfast.
  - If going out in the community to a medical test with instructions not to eat before test, pack breakfast and pills to have after test.
  - Empty CPAP water tray. Follow CPAP directions in chapter 6, "Resources," for cleaning.
- *Make bed.
- *Plan lunch and dinner.
  - Check refrigerator for leftovers or something being defrosted for dinner. Always try to use leftovers before they spoil.
  - Food taken out of freezer must be labeled with date taken out in case you don't end up cooking it that day. See section D-4 in this chapter for directions.
- *If RS is going out in the community the next day, get community ready. See chapter 5, "Community," section A.
  - Make sure medical or social community form is filled out.
  - If anything is missing on form, contact KF.
  - Check that day and time match RS Calendar entry.

- For social event, check dress code and help select clothes.
- Hang clothes on closet door.
- Plan wake-up time per section G in this chapter.
- Do not change RS thermostat.
  - If you are chilled, TM blankets are in storage bags in storage closet—use only your assigned blanket.
  - First-shifters and subs: Two bags are in closet labeled, "subs" and "first-shifters" for your use and to put in laundry after shift.
  - Blankets are washed according to chore schedule in TM Calendar.

Daytime Shift Chores: In addition to tasks on daily checklist, complete these assigned chores daily, except where indicated:

- Do laundry if laundry day. See section C in this chapter.
- Cook any defrosted foods found in refrigerator (label date food is cooked).
- Put any cooked food not consumed within two days of cooking into freezer.
- See chapter 6, "Resources," for help with cleaning instructions.
- Review TM Calendar (inside pocket of Checklist binder) for any monthly chores to be done that day.
- Clean kitchen.
- Empty bedroom waste basket.
- Sweep bedroom floor, including under the bed.
- Steam clean bedroom floor (Sunday, Tuesday, and Friday).
- Dust bedroom shelves and bureaus using microfiber cloth (Saturday).
- Use disinfectant wipes on all bedroom and closet doorknobs and wall light switch (Saturday).
  - *Take out trash and recyclables.
    - If you unpacked any boxes, flatten them to put in recycle bin.
    - Trash/recycle room is to right of laundry room.
    - Follow rules on pink card on wall 3 for briefly leaving RS alone to take out trash or recyclables.
- Once chore is completed, initial next to chore on TM Calendar.
- If unable to complete chore that day, post a team note on TM easel for next daytime shift to complete.

Section I: Overnight Shift (9:30 p.m.–9:30 a.m.)

- For details on starting and ending shifts, see chapter 1, "Introduction," section B.
- Complete daily checklist throughout the shift.
- If RS is going out in the community the next day, check that everything is community ready. See chapter 5, "Community," section A.
- Follow chart in section G in this chapter.
- Do not change RS thermostat.
  - If you are chilled, TM blankets are in storage bags in storage closet—use only your assigned blanket. ("First shifters" and subs: Two bags are in closet labeled, "subs and "first shifters'" for your use and to put in dirty laundry basket after shift.)
  - Once RS goes to bed, if you are warm, feel free to put on the fan or living room air conditioner.
  - Blankets are washed according to chore schedule in TM Calendar.

Overnight Shift Chores: In addition to tasks on daily checklist, complete these assigned chores daily, except where indicated:

- Prepare tomorrow's daily checklist (on turquoise clipboard).
  - Blank checklists are in Forms folder in black mesh basket on communication table.
  - Write tomorrow's date on top.
  - Put today's checklist in Checklist binder.
- Empty all wastebaskets except bedroom basket into one trash bag. Empty recycle basket into a separate paper bag.
  - Trash/recycle room is to right of laundry room.
  - Take out trash/recycling in morning, at end of your shift, or if RS is awake and not in bed, per rules on pink card on wall 3.
- Empty and wash water bottle and put in drying rack.
  - Before RS awakens, fill water bottle and put next to RS recliner.
- See chapter 6, "Resources, Household Directions, Cleaning Instructions."
- Use disinfectant wipes to clean RS recliner, living room chair, two dining table chairs, RS iPad, house phones, and RS cell phone.
- Use disinfectant wipes on all doorknobs and light switches except bedroom (Saturday).
- Sweep kitchen and living/dining room floors.
- Wipe bathroom sink, faucets, handicap bar, and mirror with disinfectant wipes.
- Steam clean bathroom, living room, and kitchen floors (Sunday, Tuesday, and Thursday).

- Clean toilet bowl (Sunday, Tuesday, Thursday).
- Use microfiber cloth to dust living room and dining tables, wall units (including shelves and items), TV cabinet, TV screen, and photos cabinet (Tuesday).

END OF TM CHAPTER 4

Chapter 5

Community

Section A: Definitions of Community

Definition of Medical Event

- Any medical appointment
- Hospital admission
- Medical test with or without an appointment
- Emergency room
- Home visit from OT or PT or neuropsychologist

Definition of Social Event

- Activities and/or meals inside or out of building with TM, family, or friends
- Social gatherings, such as a party, dance, wedding, or concert
- Casual plans
- Shopping
- Errands
- Activities with an organization
- Meetings

Leaving Apartment Building

- Includes medical events, social events, travel, errands, walking or sitting outside

Leaving RS Apartment but Staying Inside Apartment Building

- Includes dining room, activities, events, or visiting a neighbor

Staying Inside RS Apartment with Someone in Addition to TM or KF

- Includes visits from friends, family, and professionals

Definition of Community Ready

- Medical or social community form is filled out. See section B-1 in this chapter.
- Community bag is filled. See section B-2 in this chapter for list.
  (Not necessary if event is in RS apartment)
- Clothes have been selected and hanging on bedroom closet doorknob.

Section B: Preparation for Going Out in the Community

B-1: Team Preparation

- Check calendar as soon as possible at start of shift to know if community event is planned.
- If going to medical event, check blue Medical folder in community bag for information to ensure that
  - it includes details of time, place, and instructions such as if she cannot eat, drink, or take pills before a test or needs any other preparation; and
  - it includes paperwork such as lab slip or letter, which should be on left side of Medical folder.
- If medical community form is not filled out or information is missing, text/call KF.
- Check that community bag is ready with all items. See section B-2 below.
- Always allow plenty of time to complete tasks and to help RS get ready for the community. Being on time is very important. Add extra time for
  - getting RS ready (see section B-3 in this chapter);
  - RS slow pace of moving;
  - RS going to bathroom;
  - RS getting to and into car;
  - traffic, especially if traveling during rush hour;
  - parking, if you are driving; and
  - getting RS out of car and to event.
- If going to social event, check pink Social folder in community bag for information about event, time, place, and if anything needs to be brought to event.
  - If social community form is not filled out or information is missing, text/call KF.
  - Check dress code and weather. RS clothes for event should be hanging on the closet doorknob. Consider weather forecast or if RS decides to wear something else and adjust clothes accordingly.
  - Make sure any gift or food donation needed to be brought to event is ready.
  - Check that lunch and/or dinner is ready to be made or heated upon returning, if social event does not include a meal.

B-2: Community Bag

- Bag with "Community" luggage tag is kept under communication table.
- Luggage tag has Rayna's first name and cell number only, in case of loss.
- Community bag must always be with RS when she leaves apartment, except for the following when she only needs to take medication pouch:

- walking or sitting inside or outside apartment building
- going to building celebrations or events
- You must always bring your cell phone and take apartment lanyard (on wall 3 to right of storage closet).
- Community bag must always be stocked with items listed on next page.

List of Community Bag Contents

1. RS personal calendar (from Checklist binder pocket) and pencil (never use pen) to write in calendar

2. RS wallet with credit card, insurance card, ID, and cash for parking and/or valet tip, if credit card not allowed

3. Handicap placard

4. Tissues

5. Health history envelope

6. Filled water bottle

7. Pair of gripper socks, regular socks, extra clothing

8. RS cell phone

9. Community booklet, which includes the following:

   a. Chapter 1: Introduction

   b. Chapter 2: Medical and Safety

   c. Chapter 5: Community

   d. List of "Products Preferences, Portion and Food Guidelines"

   e. List of "Allergies and Intolerances"

10. Two nylon reusable bags, in case of any purchases

11. Blue Medical Community folder and pink Social Community folder

12. Extra gloves and masks

13. Three snacks

    a. Shaklee bar

    b. crackers or chips

    c. fruit with nuts or vegetables

14. Medication pouch

    a. Lactaid pills

    b. Tylenol pills

    c. community pill container

    d. eye treatment supplies

B-3: Rayna Preparation

Before heading out, make sure:

- RS brushes her teeth.
- RS has on arm brace (stored in bedroom on top of tall bureau).
- RS has on compression stockings (in right top drawer of bedroom multicolored bureau) and ankle brace (kept with shoes in bedroom against back wall).
- If PT/OT or anyone is coming to house, make sure RS is prepared in advance:
  - wearing ankle brace, compression stockings, shoes, arm brace, and gait belt
  - not eating
  - finished bathroom needs
  - not sleeping

B-4: Checklist of What to Bring

- Apartment lanyard
- Community bag with medical or social community form completed with address, phone number, and details
- Transport wheelchair
- RS cane
- Lunch or dinner if RS attends social event that does not include food
- Fancy handbag if RS wants for a dressy event

B-5: Car Travel Procedures

- To prevent car sickness, RS must not have an empty stomach when she travels, unless fasting for a medical test. Bring something to eat after test.
- Always bring her cane.
- Do not play any music in your car that is vulgar, sexual, with swears or violence. RS should approve music.

Getting In and Out of Car

- If weather is good, use back parking lot door to wheel RS outside to car.
- If weather is cold, rainy, or icy,
  - wheel RS to main lobby entrance;
  - have her sit inside lobby near elevators while you get your car;

- park at Passenger Loading Zone sign;
- reverse procedure when returning to apartment.
- Park transport wheelchair as close to car as possible and then lock the wheels.
- Be very careful helping RS transfer to car.
    - Notice any curb she could trip over.
    - Help RS use cane to stand and get in or out of car.
    - Make sure RS gets her body far back in the seat.
- You may have to help RS with her seat belt.
- Cue her to sit up straight when in car.
- Cue her to stand straight when exiting car, standing, or walking, to raise head, and to put shoulders back, because leaning forward could cause her to fall.

Before You Shut Car Door

- Be very careful RS right knee and arm are away from door.
- Say a verbal cue like "Knee and arm in car."
- Watch that knee and arm remain far away from door, and do not flop as you shut the door.

Parking

- If you valet or self-park, RS will use her credit card to pay. Remind her to put card back in wallet.
- If credit cards are not accepted, use designated money in RS wallet and keep receipts.
- If you park on your own, remember to hang handicap placard on rearview mirror.
- If you use valet parking, show handicap placard and inform attendant your passenger has a disability.
    - Many places waive a fee for handicap parking. If fee not waived, pay for valet and keep receipt.
    - Even if valet parking fee is waived, always tip valet (with prearranged amount according to KF).

Make sure to return handicap placard to community bag.

Section C: Procedures for Going Out in the Community and Returning Home

Using Bathroom

- RS uses her cane when not in transport wheelchair.
- Wheel RS inside bathroom and into stall if possible.
- If not possible to do so, leave wheelchair outside stall door or bathroom door and have RS use cane.
  - *Never leave personal belongings in wheelchair* unless chair is in stall with you.
- Make sure to stay with her and help while she is in bathroom.

Planned or Unexpected Shopping/Eating When Out in the Community

When out in the community or at a restaurant, getting takeout food or shopping in a store, follow these guidelines:

- Never let RS go in store alone to get takeout or to shop.
- Do not let RS sit in a booth before you check that booth table can move.
- Before ordering food, see list for "Allergies and Intolerances" in community booklet in community bag.
- RS will pay with her credit card for any of her purchases.
  - Cue her to put receipts and credit card back in wallet.
- RS has weekly spending money to use as she wants. Guide her choices. Never say "can't." Use gentle language such as, "Rayna, this is your money, but let me guide you."
- If RS wants to purchase something above her weekly amount, contact KF.
  - If you cannot reach KF, call other members on family list. (See contact list/ communications chart in chapter 2, "Medical and Safety," section A-1 in community booklet in community bag.)
  - If no KF is reached, buy it and ask for the receipt, or ask the store clerk to put the item on hold.

Social Event Food

- See list for "Allergies and Intolerances" in community booklet in community bag.

Medical Event

- When checking in, give health history form to be copied for doctor.
- Ask doctor or medical person involved in RS visit to fill out medical notes on medical community form in blue folder and include any relevant paperwork. Alternative is to get a printed appointment summary.
- If medication is prescribed, confirm with pharmacy if it will be delivered or must be picked up. Ask for it to be ready immediately if possible, so you can pick it up on your way to RS home. If not, text KF for help to pick up prescription(s).
- After appointment, help RS use bathroom before driving home.

Procedures Returning Home

- Initial and put all receipts in LTM mailbox.
- Medical
  - Call AGY/KF with report if new medicine and/or procedures.
  - Put all medical notes in KF mailbox.
  - All new medications go on dining table-TM side.
- If new medical procedure was ordered, such as elevate legs or take a medicine, fill out and post RF corkboard form. Directions for RF corkboard form are in chapter 3, "Communications," section B.
- Community bag
  - Leave, replace, or remove items per chart below:

LEAVE IN BAG	REPLACE AS NEEDED	REMOVE FROM BAG
medical pouch (with two Tylenol and Lactaid)	Lactaid and/or Tylenol if low or used up (in medical pouch)	RS cell phone
pencil	extra gloves and masks	perishable snacks
health history envelope	tissues	water bottle
blue and pink folders	Shaklee bar	RS Calendar
handicap placard	extra clothing, underpants, or regular socks and gripper socks	paperwork, parking and/or shopping receipts—put in LTM mailbox.
community booklet	two nylon reusable bags	extra clothing if used
RS wallet with credit card, insurance card, ID, and cash	cash in wallet—leave message for LTM to replace.	

END OF TM CHAPTER 5

Chapter 6

Resources

Author Note: Chapter 6 includes directions, charts, lists, and forms. The full list is below, followed by a few samples of forms I created. This is what the table of contents would look like in the Resources chapter of Rayna's Team Member Handbook.

DAILY CHECKLIST

DATE:_____   *TM: Initial each task when done*

Explanation of tasks in chapter 1, "Introduction," section F
Checklist is on front and back

Morning/Afternoon	Initial	Afternoon/Evening	Initial
Meals planned for the day		PT/OT exercises or PT/OT session if not in a.m.	
Brush teeth		Positive activities #	
Brush hair		Walk routes if not in a.m.	
Shower or sponge bath (alternate days). Circle one.		Outside 10+ minutes if not in a.m.	
Skin creams		Community ready if not in a.m.	
Wearing second-day clothes		Laundry (when shower or as needed)	
Eye treatment		Cue pills 7:00 p.m.	
Clean eyeglasses		Eye treatment	
Mouth guard soak		Brush teeth	
Cue pills with food in morning		Prescription mouthwash (Wednesday)	
CPAP morning cleaning		Brush hair and leave loose	
PT/OT exercises or PT/OT session		Fill CPAP with distilled water	
Walk routes		Bedtime essentials	
Outside for 10+ minutes		Charge RS cell phone	
Positive activities #_____		Clean ankle brace	
Community ready		Apartment chores completed	
Laundry (shower day or as needed)			

TURN OVER FOR ADDITIONAL DAILY CHECKLIST TASKS

DAILY CHECKLIST

DATE:_____   *TM: Initial each task when done*

Circle when completed:

Sit/stand exercise: 1 2 3 4 5   **Arm exercises:** 1 2 3   **Water bottles:** 1 2 3

Positive activities: **Gratitude**   **Music**

Headspace or Calm   **Ted Talks or Lumosity**   **Game or Crafts or Cook**

Time	SCHEDULED TASKS—Circle each task when completed and initial	Initial
10:00 a.m.	**Gait Belt ON** **Compression Stockings/Ankle Brace ON** **Arm Brace ON** **TheraTears** **Reposition**	
12:00 p.m.	**TheraTears** **Reposition**	
2:00 p.m.	**TheraTears** **Reposition**	
4:00 p.m.	**TheraTears** **Reposition** **Compression Stockings/Ankle Brace OFF**	
6:00 p.m.	**TheraTears** **Reposition** **Compression Stockings/Ankle Brace ON**	
8:00 p.m.	**TheraTears** **Reposition**	
10:00 p.m.	**Gait Belt OFF** **Compression Stockings/Ankle Brace OFF** **Arm Brace OFF**	
Overnight	**Chores completed**	

Sandy Tovray Greenberg

LAUNDRY SIGN-OUT FORM

Date	TM	Amount Start	Amount Finished	Initial That You Returned Card

MEDICINE/FEVER FORM

Date	TM Initial	Illness	Medicine	Time Given	Temp: Time taken: If fever, take 2 hours later. If goes up, call doctor.	Progress Notes
					Temp: Time taken:	
					Temp: Time taken:	
					Temp: Time taken:	
					Temp: Time taken:	
					Temp: Time taken:	
					Temp: Time taken:	
					Temp: Time taken:	

When page is full, if RS still sick, start another sheet and put full one underneath so you can look back for information. *Never* throw out a sheet. When notified RS is well, put sheets in LTM mailbox.

RF CORKBOARD FORM—FRONT

Date:_____ TM:_____

Red Flag situation: _____

Complete medicine/fever chart if RS has a fever and/or if she is taking medication. Place on red clipboard and leave on dining table-TM side. Front is for medical. Back is for emotional (and additional medical information if needed).

If new medicine, name of medicine_____

Time of first dose? _____ How many times a day? _____

How many days? _____

Take medicine with food or empty stomach? _____

Did doctor discontinue a medicine that is in pill container? YES_____ NO____

If YES, what is medicine? _____

If YES, tape a note on top of pill container NOT to give RS that pill until KF can remove it and send a text to all TM.

CRUCIAL: When you give RS a new medication, be aware of possible allergic reactions, and don't leave her alone. (If pill is at bedtime, sit in her room).

Print initials to confirm you read this RF Corkboard Form—Front:

_____ _____ _____ _____ _____ _____ _____ _____

Turn form over to read back

RF CORKBOARD FORM—BACK

Please print clearly

_____

_____

_____

_____

_____

_____

_____

_____

_____

_____

_____

_____

Print initials to confirm you read this RF Corkboard Form—Back:

_____ _____ _____ _____ _____ _____ _____ _____

SHIFT IN/OUT LIST

STARTING SHIFTS

- Tape TM contact card to left arm of RS recliner.
- Check cork/whiteboard and red clipboard with medicine/fever form if on dining table.
- Review daily checklist.
- Review Checklist binder calendar.
- Review past daily checklists since your last shift (first-shifters go back three days).
- Check TM easel for team notes.
- Check TM mailbox for messages.
- Determine if laundry needs to be done on your shift.

ENDING SHIFTS

- Check all areas on floor are clear.
- Initial all completed tasks on daily checklist.
- Remove TM contact card from RS recliner and return to side table basket.
- If applicable on your shift,
  - write and post corkboard red flag form for urgent communications;
  - post team note(s) on TM easel;
  - write on RS fever/medication form if RS is sick;
  - write date on food if taken out of freezer;
  - label cooked food or leftovers with date;
  - enter RS meals and snacks in food calendar in Food/Recipe binder;
  - clean dishes;
  - refill community bag if used anything in bag/medical pouch;
  - put messages in LTM mailbox; and
  - return lanyard to hook.
- Make sure RS goes to the bathroom before you leave.
- Make sure to say good-bye to RS when you leave.

Reminder: You cannot leave until next shift arrives.

Initial: _____ _____ _____

TEAM NOTES

DATE:_____ **TO:**_____ **FROM:**_____

_____

_____

_____

_____

_____

_____

TM Initial who wrote note:_____ **TM Initial when read:** _____ _____ _____ _____

- -

TEAM NOTES

DATE:_____ **TO:**_____ **FROM:**_____

_____

_____

_____

_____

_____

_____

TM Initial who wrote note:_____ **TM Initial when read:** _____ _____ _____ _____

TRANSPORT WHEELCHAIR CHART

- Transport Wheelchair Chart lists facilities with wheelchairs where you can leave RS transport wheelchair in car.
- Always take RS cane.
- Once at location, RS may want to stay in transport/wheelchair or sit in a regular chair.

Use transport wheelchair	Transport wheelchair may be left in car
All doctors' appointments not at hospital	All hospital visits
Any outdoor activity or event	Therapeutic massage
Any mall and grocery shopping	Mother's house

END OF TM CHAPTER 6

Part Four

Rayna's Lead Team Member Handbook: Sample

CONTENTS

Author Note: This is where you would put the table of contents with corresponding page numbers for your handbook.

Chapter 1

LTM Calendars

Section A: Overview

Section B: LTM Annual Calendar

Section C: RS Calendar

Section D: TM Calendar

Section A: Overview

LTM oversees three calendars:

- LTM Annual Calendar
- RS Calendar
- TM Calendar

KF purchases the calendars for upcoming new year as early as possible, even in September.

Section B: LTM Annual Calendar

LTM annual calendar is more of an annual list to assure that all tasks and all annual medical and social events are documented. Some will need to be scheduled, and some will already be booked, such as an annual medical appointment that is booked for the following year. LTM works off this annual list to add and update RS Calendar and TM Calendar for the coming year.

Regularly Scheduled Medical Events (or as needed)

- eye exam—annual
- physical—annual
- gynecology—annual
- mammogram—annual
- dermatology—annual
- flu shot—annual
  - always close to September
  - administered at pharmacy or doctor's office
- neurology—annual
- pulmonary—every six months
- tetanus shot—according to schedule. See health history form for latest update.
- colonoscopy
  - Initiate at age forty-five or when doctor advises.
- pneumococcal and shingles vaccinations
  - RS doctor will advise when needed.

Social Events

- Meetings such as monthly support group for Brain Injury Alliance of CT (BIACT)
- Activities and celebrations from RS AGY, apartment building, or out in the community
- Miscellaneous social events and appointments, such as
  - haircut
  - trip to favorite apple orchard in the fall

LTM Ongoing Responsibilities/Tasks

Some tasks are reserved only for LTM to complete because of nature of task. If TM can complete task, "*TM" is next to task.

Every Shift

- If RF (red flag) corkboard note is posted, convert to RF list.
- Check LTM mailbox and address any messages.
- Check RS mailbox in lobby.
- Clean eyeglasses. *TM. See TM chapter 4, section B-4.
- Water plants if applicable. *TM. Watering schedule is in notes section at back of TM calendar.
- Check that overnight *TM chores were completed.

Overnight *TM Chore List

- Empty wastebaskets (except in RS bedroom).
- Clean stove burners, if needed.
- Clean oven, if needed.
- Wipe shelves in refrigerator.
- Clean bathroom.
- Clean living room floors.

Weekly

Monday

- Go through Birthday/Anniversary Chart in back of TM calendar for the current week and the next week for people RS to call, text, Facebook, buy or make a card or gift to give in person or mail—whatever RS wants to do. Have her choose one or a combination of above alternatives.
- Wash sheets. *TM

Tuesday

- Dust wall unit shelves and all other living room surfaces. *TM

Wednesday

- Review inventory and shop for groceries.

Thursday

- Prepare for weekend TM:
  - money on laundry card
  - detergent stocked for laundry
  - refrigerator stocked for food
  - If social/medical appointments, make sure community forms are filled out and contact weekend TM to remind about weekend social plans/appointments.

Friday

- If new social plan or medical event came up, fill out community form(s).
- Leave messages about information and/or instructions for weekend TM.

Semimonthly

- Replace CPAP filter.

Monthly

- Wash overnight TM blankets. *TM
- Charge RS Life Alert 911 button. *TM. See TM chapter 6, "Resources."
- Clean brushes/combs. *TM. See TM chapter 4, "Daily Procedures," section B-4.
- Print forms needed for ongoing communications.
- Remove daily checklists from Checklist binder and put in KF mailbox. Leave last three days of the old month in binder.
- Prepare order to Shaklee.
- Review Amazon Subscribe and Save.
- Scan medical visits and reports into computer. Also, e-mail them to KF.
- Review CPAP instructions for other timely updates of accessories.

Quarterly (weeks of January 1, April 1, July 1, and October 1)

- Replace toothbrush.
    - Replace after RS has been sick and readjust quarterly schedule in TM calendar.
- Wash RS comforter, pillows. *TM. See TM chapter 4, "Daily Procedures," section C.
- Wash TM blankets. *TM. See TM chapter 4, "Daily Procedures," section C.
    - Read washing instructions on blankets, comforters, and pillows.

Section C: RS Calendar

A one-year calendar is always used with notes in the back to write any medical appointments and social events scheduled for the upcoming year. These will be transferred to the new calendar once it is purchased. Examples:

- RS has an annual checkup at dermatologist, and appointment is made for the following year.
- RS gets a save-the-date announcement for an event to happen the following year.

Although all TM write in current RS Calendar as needed when they are on shift, LTM sets up RS Calendar for the upcoming new year.

Setting up RS Calendar for Upcoming New Year

- Create a large label, "RS Calendar," and attach label to front of calendar.
- Fill in all ongoing social events from section B in this chapter, such as a monthly support group.
- Transfer any medical and social events scheduled for the new year (listed in the back of old calendar).

Section D: TM Calendar

Setting up TM Calendar

- Create a large label, "TM Calendar," and attach label to front of calendar.
- By January (preferably before), fill in all items on LTM Annual Calendar from section B in this chapter.
- If directions are needed to complete *TM task, LTM includes where to find that information in the calendar.
  - Example: Clean brushes/combs *TM. See TM chapter 4, "Daily Procedures," section B-4.
- Overnight shift is responsible to check TM Calendar to see if a task needs to be completed for the next day shift.
  - If there is a task, overnight shift fills out a team note describing the task and posts it on TM easel.
  - When TM completes task, she initials the team note and puts it in LTM mailbox.

END OF LTM CHAPTER 1

Chapter 2

LTM Communication

In addition to the LTM Calendar, LTM keeps separate communication tools, including a notebook for LTM task reminders and a file folder for LTM forms.

LTM Communication Responsibilities

- Communicate with TM, KF, and AGY.
- Help RS with correspondence, such as postal mail, e-mails, texts, invitations.
- Oversee that social and medical scheduling is being completed properly in the calendar.
- Create community and medical forms to put in folders.
- Write a newsletter (KF option).
- Oversee red flag situations.
- Manage messages in LTM mailbox.
- Keep an LTM notebook for all tasks beyond TM responsibilities.

LTM Notebook

LTM keeps a notebook to track responsibilities beyond those listed in LTM Chapter 1. These include:

- Tasks requested by KF, such as to book an appointment with a new doctor.
- Tasks initiated on LTM shift that cannot be completed on her shift. Examples:
  - LTM took RS to a doctor who asked for a callback the next day with an update on RS condition and LTM is not on shift that day, so TM needs to make the call.
  - Tasks such as a situation when RS gets a call at night with an invitation to dinner the next day and wants to bring a dessert. LTM needs TM on the next day shift to help RS make or buy a dessert.

Red Flag (RF) Situations

If LTM comes to shift and sees an RF corkboard form posted, see TM handbook chapter 3, "Communication," section B, and follow these steps:

- Copy the information onto the whiteboard side, and in addition, copy it on an RF list to track the red flag situation. See RF list in next chapter, chapter 3, "LTM Resources."
- Remove RF corkboard form and recycle it.
- Track situation on RF list as well as write updates on whiteboard side of cork/whiteboard.
- Continue tracking and writing updates until situation is resolved or under control with a plan in place if needed, such as RS healing from grief or a pandemic.
  - Revisit, if needed, RF list and update TM if situation under control reverses.
- If RF situations happen on LTM shift, RF corkboard form is not necessary. LTM starts an RF list and writes RF information on whiteboard side of cork/whiteboard.

END OF LTM CHAPTER 2

Chapter 3

LTM Resources

In addition to TM resources, LTM has a set of directions, charts, lists, and forms.

Like chapter 6, "Resources," in TM handbook, I created forms and lists and included these in this chapter:

1. Medical community form
2. Social community form
3. RF list

Medical Community Form and Social Community Form

LTM fills out these forms after she schedules and enters a new event on the calendar or gets a message form in her mailbox about a new calendar entry so that TM and substitutes have all pertinent information to take RS in the community.

- Forms for social or medical scheduled events are in community bag.
- Medical events are in blue folder; social in pink folder.
- Forms are placed on the clipboard on right side of folder.
- Left side of Medical folder is for any paper, lab or test slips needed for RS appointment.
- For medical: Space is provided on front and back for doctor to write notes.
    - Alternative: Office provides printed summary of visit.
- When LTM finds a medical community form or printed summary of visit in LTM mailbox, she scans information into computer and e-mails summary to AGY/KF.
    - If any new information about a medical visit, such as a change in medication or a procedure to follow (like icing an injury), fill out an RF corkboard form, and also text AGY.
- TM are instructed they will not need forms for specified events in calendar such as

- events in apartment building, and
- friend or family visiting.

Optional

Create standard forms for social and medical for recurring social and medical events. Example: monthly Brain Injury Alliance of CT support group.

- To accomplish this, LTM
  - fills out social community form;
  - permanently leaves form on left side of folder in a plastic sleeve.
- When recurring event has a temporary change of location, day, or time, LTM
  - copies standard recurring form;
  - removes standard recurring form and puts it in her LTM File Folder;
  - edits particulars needing the change and writes, "Temporary" on top of edited form;
  - puts temporary form on right side of clipboard;
  - discards temporary form after event;
  - returns recurring form from LTM File Folder to left side.
- If temporary recurring event should become permanent, such as temporary time change is now the new time of event, LTM
  - edits recurring form with new information;
  - discards old recurring form;
  - places new recurring form inside plastic sleeve and leaves on left side of folder.

MEDICAL COMMUNITY FORM

LTM/TM initial that you wrote appointment in calendar	
LTM/TM initial who took RS to medical	

Fill in name of doctor, testing location, or other medical related information, such as shoe store for orthopedic shoes or a place to get brace adjusted.

Name of doctor and/or facility: _____

Date: _____ Time: _____ Phone: _____

Street: _____ Town: _____

Does RS need to bring anything? List here:

_____

If RS needs to bring any documents, put them in the pocket on the left side of this folder, or if already there, make sure to take the papers in to the appointment or test. The needed document(s) might be in an envelope with the contents written across the front.

If RS is having a blood test or any kind of test, can she eat before, or is there special preparation for test? YES_____ NO_____ If yes, explain: _____

What time do you need to leave? _____

Use GPS to get miles and travel time. (Before leaving, add extra time to allow for delays caused by traffic, RS moving slowly, and bathroom visits.)

Do you need transport wheelchair inside the facility? YES___ NO_____ (see TM chapter 6, "Resources")

If this is a test or shot, read the laminated instructions in the big pocket on the left side of this folder labeled "Medical Tests, Shots, and Blood Tests." (Instructions list helpful suggestions to best take RS blood, etc.)

Ask doctor to write notes about appointment on back of sheet or get an appointment printout.

SOCIAL COMMUNITY FORM

LTM/TM initial that you wrote event in calendar	
LTM/TM initial who took RS to event	

Date of event: _____ Time of event: _____

Event: _____

Copy details from the invite and leave in LTM mailbox. If phone call, also leave message form in LTM mailbox.

Person or organization hosting event: _____

Street: _____ Town: _____

Phone number if available: _____

What time do you need to leave? _____

Use GPS to get miles and travel time. (Before leaving, add extra time to allow for delays caused by traffic, RS moving slowly, and bathroom visits.)

Do you need transport wheelchair at event? YES____ NO____ (see TM chapter 6, "Resources")

Check if dress code on invitation. Discuss outfits with RS and KF.

Dressy_____ Casual_____ No dress code_____ Outdoor event? YES___ NO___

(On day of event, make sure outfit matches that day's weather.)

If can't determine if event is outdoor from invitation, call number on invitation or flyer or put message form with question in LTM mailbox or call KF if event on same day.

Does RS need to bring anything? If yes, fill in next line. YES_____ NO_____

Gift? Grab bag? Food bank donation? Food for potluck meal? _____

Put message form about what RS needs in LTM mailbox.

RED FLAG LIST

Date	Red Flag Situation	Initial	Updates	Initial	Completed

Circle any RF event not resolved and copy onto next page.

Part Five

Rayna's Key Family Handbook:
Sample

CONTENTS

Author Note: This is where you would put the table of contents with corresponding page numbers for your handbook.

Chapter 1

KF Calendars

KF buys two calendars a year: one is for RS appointments and social events and one for TM to indicate chores from LTM Annual Calendar. See LTM handbook chapter 1, section B.

- RS Calendar must be a spiral bound eight-by-ten desk calendar to fit into community bag and have a place for notes on the back.
- TM Calendar can be a wall calendar because it stays in the apartment.
- Both calendars must be a one-year-only calendar. Do not buy an eighteen-month or two-year calendar, etc.
- Before January of each year, work with LTM to update LTM Annual Calendar to make sure each item on the list is completed for the year.
- Insert copy of updated Birthday/Anniversary Chart in back of RS calendar before giving calendar to TM.

BIRTHDAY/ANNIVERSARY CHART

Name	Date	Birthday or Anniversary	Phone number	E-Mail	Notes/relation (e.g., family, friend)

Outside Help

Four times a year, January, April, July, October, hire outside help for a deep cleaning of RS apartment, to include the following:

- Clean windows.
- Clean window blinds.
- Clean oven.
- Rotate and flip mattress.
- Replace A/C filter.
- Move furniture, bed, and refrigerator away from wall to clean behind.

END OF KF CHAPTER 1

Chapter 2

KF Finances and Passwords

Finances

KF manages all financials and chooses certain financial responsibilities, if any, for LTM, such as arranging cash for RS home to allow LTM to cover petty cash such as money on a laundry card for apartment washer and dryer.

Suggestions include the following:

- Deliver cash to home on a set date or as needed.
- Set up a prepaid card. KF controls how much cash to put on card.
- Set up a small checking account.
    - Set up account online.
    - Link account to your checking account.
    - Transfer small amounts of cash and oversee account.

No matter which suggestion you choose, it is best to

- devise a manner to lock up cash and banking passwords in a secure place;
- use, if possible, locks with codes, which can be changed easily if needed, rather than keys;
- verbally give account passcode to LTM; and
- request written tally of expenses.

KF can also request LTM to contact KF for directions when RS receives checks or cash, such as from rebates and gifts.

Passwords

KF can coordinate passwords for LTM.

KF keeps written account of all passwords and uses her discretion what to share with LTM.

- KF instructs LTM to lock up passwords, never save them on any RS electronic devices, and always log out.

END OF KF CHAPTER 2

Chapter 3

KF Annual Renewals and Recertifications

KF oversees all annual rebates, renewals, and recertifications, such as rental insurance, town rental rebate, Department of Social Services (DSS), Housing and Urban Development (HUD).

- KF requests notification by LTM of any correspondence regarding rebates, renewals, and recertifications.
- KF requests that LTM provide supporting documents when applicable, such as receipts.
- KF keeps copy of each renewal and recertification.
- KF replaces copies and discards when
  - submissions are acted upon, such as rebate issued; and
  - updated renewals, and recertifications are issued.

END OF KF CHAPTER 3

Chapter 4

KF Updating RS Information

Repeated Topics

All changes in RS life (e.g., routines, schedules, health information) must be updated. It is crucial to assure updates are made in every area. All updates need to be shared between LTM and KF. Places that can be affected by updates include the following:

- Any or all handbooks
- Community booklet
- Orientation sheet
- Papers posted on the walls
- Contact names, numbers, and address book
- Many directives and information repeat in a few chapters because they apply to more than one topic.
  - Example: Rules for leaving RS alone in apartment are in three places:
    - In TM chapter 2, "Medical and Safety," section B-1
    - In TM chapter 6, "Resources"
    - Posted on a pink card on wall 3

Steps for Handbook

- Check if new edits throw off alignment, and if so, realign accordingly.
- Print new page(s) and recycle old information.
- Print a copy of edited page(s) and highlight new information; attach the new pages to a message form in TM mailbox stating changes including an initial strip at bottom of message.
- Follow repeated directives procedures.
  - Each time information is edited in any of the handbooks, new information must be put in all places with a change.

Contacts Box

- All information in contacts box includes the following:
  - KF
  - Social worker
  - Neuropsychologist
  - Apartment building personnel
  - Friends and family
  - Businesses
  - Organizations
  - All doctors, medical facilities, and equipment facilities
    - If a group practice, update name of RS main doctor.
- Do not cross out old information to update.
  - Rewrite a new card.
  - Toss out old contact.

Medical Information

- Medical history needs to be updated in both the handbook and the health history form that is always in an envelope in the community bag.
- KF instructs LTM to be notified of all health updates.
- KF puts all updates into health history form.
- KF e-mails new health history form to LTM, and requests that
  - LTM prints out two copies and keeps one in Master Forms folder and puts other in plastic envelope in RS community bag.
  - LTM makes sure to shred old medical history.
  - LTM does not include any personal, sensitive information such as RS full name and address on health history in case community bag is lost. LTM offers that information to doctor verbally and contacts KF if any questions.
- Updates also include changes in pills, allergies, and intolerances, CPAP machine, PT/OT, or any medical, emotional, or cognitive changes, etc.

Pill List and Pill Container

Update pill list in two places:

- Health history form
- TM handbook (chapter 6, "Resources")

Update pill container

- Remove old pills from main pill container and backup tray.
- Put message form with pill change and initial strip in TM mailbox.

Community Bag

- Change information on luggage tag on community bag.
- Add, delete, or change any contents.

Birthday/Anniversary List

- Update as needed

Inventory List for Food and Supplies

- Orders from Internet: Amazon, Shaklee, etc.
- Update product preferences, portion, and food guidelines.

END OF KF CHAPTER 4

Chapter 5

KF Travel and Packing

Section A: Time Frame Prior to Travel

A-1: As Soon as Possible

Traveler(s) Accompanying RS

- As soon as travel dates are confirmed, contact AGY/LTM. Even if you are traveling with RS and TM, KF coordinates with LTM all travel arrangements.
  - Give dates of travel.
  - Gather all information about travel companion(s) for booking tickets, such as legal name, address, and phone number.

Book Ticket

- Book immediately when plans are confirmed.
- If airlines have not opened booking dates, find out when dates open and put in calendar to book immediately.
- Always call airline. Never book online.
- Request to speak to someone about special assistance for disability.
  - State you are booking tickets for a traveler with a disability and an aide, and, if applicable, anyone else traveling with RS.
  - Choosing seats: Always request a first row and on left aisle as you enter the airplane, so RS left hand is on an aisle. Book seats for aide and anyone else traveling to sit next to her. If not possible, book for aide to sit next to her.
  - You can explain to booking agent that RS right side is partially paralyzed and sometimes drops down, and as passengers walk by her seat, they can bump her arm.
- Arrange transportation to and from airport.
- Fill out travel questionnaire on next page to help with packing.

Travel Questionnaire

Destination: _____

Date of departure: _____

Date of return trip: _____

Total number of days she will be away: _____

Will she have access to washer and dryer? _____

What is the weather forecast at her destination? _____

Weather forecast for leaving: _____

Weather forecast for returning: _____

Is this a formal event? _____ If yes, see formal event at end of standard travel list.

A-2: Two Weeks before Travel

- Plan food shopping list with LTM:
  - Stop buying perishables that won't get used prior to travel.
  - Measure amount. Example: Don't buy a new milk that will go bad while RS is away.
  - If need be, adjust amount; buy one quart rather than half gallon.
  - Buy snacks of nuts, chips, or crackers in individual packages.
  - If driving, buy a bottle of distilled water for CPAP machine. If flying, buy it at the destination.

A-3: One Week before Travel

- Print packing list so TM or LTM can help RS cross off as packing happens. See section D in this chapter for the packing list.
- Start packing (all travel bags are in storage closet).
- Make sure RS has one-dollar bills for tipping if she engages a porter for assistance. She needs at least ten ones.
- Always pack medicines for two days more than she is traveling in case of delays coming home.

- If no one is available to check mail and travel is more than two nights, arrange to hold mail at post office.

A-4: One Day before Travel

- Check weather forecast and adjust packing accordingly.
- Make sure all items on packing list are completed.
- Check RS into airlines and print boarding pass.
  - Put printed boarding pass on outside zippered pocket of community bag.
  - Also put boarding pass on her cell.
- Confirm transportation to and from airport.
- Clean out refrigerator of perishables.
- Put all luggage together in one area behind RS recliner chair.

Section B: Day of Travel

- If flying,
  - leave for airport according to airline guidelines regarding time to arrive;
  - check GPS for travel time;
  - add thirty minutes to travel time for RS to get in and out of car and possible longer bathroom time; and
  - have RS go to bathroom before leaving.
- Put last-minute items in community bag. Add community bag to other bags. See section D for list of items you need to add and those you can leave at home.
- Pack CPAP. See section D. Add CPAP to other luggage.
- Count number of bags.
- Take cane.
- Shut all shades and lights.
- Do not use handicap button to close apartment building door. Open the door manually, so it shuts quicker.
  - Watch that it shuts.

Section C: Returning Home

- Depending on time of arrival and availability for help, restock refrigerator.
- Unpack as soon as possible.
- Remove travel items in community bag and replace with items you took out for travel.
- If stopped mail, pick up at post office.
- Return suitcase(s), CPAP travel bag, and carry-on bag to storage closet.

Section D: Packing List

In addition to suitcase(s), RS should have two carry-on bags.

Community bag: notes below

CPAP machine: notes below

Community Bag

Remove from community bag and leave these items on dining table-TM side and put a note on top, "Return to Community Bag After Travel":

- RS calendar
- blue and pink folders

Add to community bag for travel: (put liquids and sprays in small Ziplock bag)

- daily pills for length of time plus extra for two days
- fresh snacks
- empty, clean water bottle
- tickets
- cell phone and charger
- iPad and charger
- earplugs and eye mask
- eye treatment medicine
- nighttime mouth guard
- nasal spray
- fine jewelry, if applicable

CPAP Machine Notes

- Always take CPAP when traveling, even for one night.
- If flying, never check CPAP in baggage.
  - Airlines do not include CPAP machine in counting maximum carry-on items.
- CPAP travel bag is in storage closet.
- Follow directions on CPAP travel bag for packing CPAP on day of travel.
- Must continue to use distilled water for CPAP machine.

- If driving, take bottle and bring home unused water.
- If flying, buy water bottle upon arrival and leave unused water at host's house or hotel.
  - If Dad's house, he will provide water bottle.

Suitcase

- Amounts to pack will vary depending on answers to travel questionnaire.
- List below is minimum amount for a trip only if a washer and dryer is at destination.

Packing List

Clothing

- 2 pjs/nightgowns
- 2 pants
- 2 capris, if applicable
- 2 shorts, if applicable
- 4 tops/tanks
- 1 dressy top
- 1 sweatshirt
- 1 sweater/light jacket depending on climate
- 3 bras
- 2 bathing suits
- 2 gripper socks
- 2 regular socks
- casual jewelry
- compression stockings; at least 4
- extra pair of shoes and/or sandals

Toiletries/medicines

- shampoo
- conditioner
- hairbrush, comb, and hair accessories
- body creams
- deodorant
- sunscreen
- toothbrush

- toothpaste
- dental floss
- mouthwash
- weekly mouth rinse
- alcohol wipes for ankle brace (in a separate plastic bag)

Formal Event

- outfit for event, usually a dressy dress
- backup outfit—for event (either another dressy dress or dressy pants and top)
- gift if occasion necessitates. Unless driving, best to buy a gift certificate rather than a package. Or mail gift ahead of time.
- dressy shoes
- dressy purse
- fine jewelry
- dressy cover-up, sweater, or jacket

END OF KF CHAPTER 5

One Last Creation

If you need an LTM and/or a KF handbook, once handbooks are completed, an option of merging handbooks can be very helpful. Onsite or offsite, a combined handbook makes it easier to have all information in one place, allowing your LTM and/or KF to have access to one complete handbook rather than flipping back and forth from books.

Thus, in the end,

- TM has a handbook for TM responsibilities;
- LTM has a handbook for TM and LTM responsibilities;
- KF has a handbook for TM, LTM and KF responsibilities.

Final Message from the Author

I hope this book has helped you start your journey to create a handbook for caregivers. I have shared stories, ideas, instructions, and my heart. I hope the sample chapters help as a reference. You might discover your own methods and ideas, or maybe even notice an area I never addressed. Find your own "I didn't know what I didn't know!" Remember my words, that a handbook is never truly finished. Even after this book went to print, more changes happened in Rayna's life. So just as life is a work in progress, so is your handbook.

While our need for caregivers might not be the same, the common thread remains: A handbook of how to take care of your loved one is a true validation of our loved one's life, no matter the age or the reason for needing outside help.

We are a community. Let's stay connected! If you follow me on Facebook or Instagram, and/or add your name to our mailing list (go to www.sandygreenbergauthor.com) you won't miss updates and events. Stay tuned for the new edition of *When God Comes Knocking*, my memoir about how our family found hope and courage during the early years of Rayna's life and discovery of her illness.

Always keep in mind, you may turn over the reins to a caregiver, but you can always adjust them along the journey.

Printed in the United States
by Baker & Taylor Publisher Services